GW01071791

KETO DIET & INTERMITTENT FASTING

2-in-1 Book

Burn Fat Like Crazy While Eating Delicious Food Going Keto + The Proven Wonders of Intermittent Fasting to Achieve That Body You've Always Wanted

MAGIC KETO: WHY IT IS CELEBRITIES' FAVORITE DIET?

Embrace The Low-Carb Lifestyle, Eat Exquisite Meals, Burn Fat Like Crazy and Experience Unbelievable Changes in Your Body in Just 30 Days

Table of Contents

Introduction

Congratulations on purchasing this book and thank you for doing so!

The following chapters will discuss what the Ketogenic Diet is and how women can get the best results out of the diet. We will go over what constitutes good fats and bad fats, how to calculate your macros, and how to overcome common mistakes made on this diet. The information found in this audiobook will best explore the adaptations a woman needs to make in order to successfully attain the metabolic state of Ketosis.

Thanks again for choosing this obook! Every effort was made to ensure it is full of as much useful information as possible. Please enjoy!

Chapter 1: What Is the Ketogenic Diet, and How Does It Work?

The Ketogenic diet (Keto, for short) is a diet that heavily reduces the number of carbohydrates (carbs) a body takes in and replaces it with fat. This low-carb, high-fat diet has been studied and has shown to help people lose weight and improve health. There are many different forms of the diet, but the standard Ketogenic diet (SKD) is the most studied and the most widely used. This diet forces the body to burn the intake of fat instead of carbohydrates.

This is how the diet works. If you were to eat a meal rich in carbs, the natural body process would take these carbs and turn them into glucose. Glucose is a sugar that is made to be a primary source of energy to all living things. It is also an integral part of a carbohydrate. Insulin is then produced to move that glucose into the bloodstream to burn for energy or body fuel. Insulin is a hormone produced by the pancreas to regulate and control how much glucose is in the bloodstream. Hence, not having enough insulin causes a form of diabetes.

On the Keto diet, things change. While the process stays the same, the carb intake is very low. Consequently, the body has to utilize another form of energy—and that is where the high-fat part of the diet comes into play. To replace the loss of carbs in the body, the liver takes the fats and turns them into Ketones as its source of energy.

Ketones and Ketosis

Ketones are now byproducts of the body breaking down fat for energy when the carb intake is low. Technically, there are three types of Ketones the body uses on the Keto diet. Acetoacetate is the first Ketone created when the body begins to break down the fat instead of carbohydrates. Acetoacetate is simply created from the process of burning fatty acids. It acts as a taxi or shuttle bus to push the body into Ketosis—much like the beta-hydroxybutyric Ketone. The acetoacetate Ketones form either the beta-hydroxybutyric Ketone or the acetone

Ketone. The beta-hydroxybutyric Ketone (BHB) is not quite a Ketone, but for the sake of the Keto diet, it is considered one. BHB is the most bountiful Ketone in the body, making up over 70% of Ketones in the blood during Ketosis. Here is where we start to see the benefits of the Ketogenic diet—but we will get into those in a bit. While acetone is the simplest Ketone produced from acetoacetate, it is the least abundant. Because BHB is so plentiful, acetone is hardly used as a source of energy. Thus, the body gets rid of it by breaking it down as waste. If a person's body is not using its acetone Ketones to produce energy, you can usually tell by an odor change in the urine or breath. The more a person's breath smells like acetone, the further into Ketosis they are.

Ketosis is a metabolic state formed from raised levels of Ketones in the body. It begins when the body starts to turn its preferred method of using glucose to exert energy to using fatty acids. There are a number of ways to tell if the body is in full Ketosis. The first one is bad breath, which we've already touched on a bit. The acetone Ketones that aren't being used to create fuel for the body are discarded through a person's breath and urine. The most noticeable change is weight loss. The Keto diet rapidly changes the body because the body needs the energy to keep going regardless of what process is being followed. Carbs retain a lot of water—once they nearly disappear from the body, so does a lot of water weight. In consequence, most people in Ketosis see weight changes within the first week. Another way to tell if the body is in Ketosis is having digestive issues. Although these side effects are short-lived while the body adapts to its new course, constipation and diarrhea are pretty common among Keto dieters.

Differences Between the Ketogenic Diet and the Atkins Diet

If you're looking to follow a low-carb diet, both the Ketogenic diet and Atkins diet rank as the most popular. The results are almost identical at first, but the Ketogenic diet began for a completely different reason. It has only recently been used for a weight-loss alternative. The methods behind the diets also differ quite a bit.

The history of the Atkins diet starts off with the founder, Robert C. Atkins. In the 1950s, after receiving his M.D., Atkins started his own practice after a growing concern of prescribed medication as appetite suppressants. The idea of giving medicine to a person to curb their hunger didn't sit well with him. So, he thought of alternative methods. He spent the next decade researching nutrition and carb intake instead of calorie counting, which was a common way of losing weight during the time. He noticed a similarity in reports of the calorie-counting, weight loss method leaving people still feeling hungry. He started a low-carb diet, himself. After noticing a difference, he then had 65 associates go through the same process, all which resulted in weight loss.

The Atkins diet is arranged into four different phases. Phases one is the induction phase—the phase that kicks off the process. The first part of the diet restricts carb intake to less than twenty grams per day while keeping protein and fat input high. Phase two introduces more carbs (between twenty and fifty grams per day). It also suggests more variety of foods, such as more berries, nuts, and vegetables. This is known as the on-going weight loss phase. Phase three is the pre-maintenance stage. It slowly allows a person to add more good carbs to the diet until they become comfortable with the rate at which they are losing weight. And finally, there is the maintenance phase. This is the stage in which the person pursuing the diet reaches their weight loss goal. They only take in the number of carbs that allows them to maintain their weight.

While the Atkins diet results in similar weight loss as the Keto diet, Keto is less structured and easier to follow. Originally, the Keto diet was introduced in the 1910s as a way to control epileptic seizures. It became more popular in the 1920s. The intermitted fasting proved effective as epilepsy therapy. The diet and fasting techniques exhausted certain toxins in the body that researchers believed caused the seizures. The diet became less commonly used with the increased productivity of medications and other sorts of therapy.

The Keto diet revolves around the idea of what the earliest humans would have put into their bodies as food sources. Some would argue that the earliest human's bodies were in a constant state of

Ketosis because of the seasonal food that was readily available to them. There were also states of natural fasting because of the lack of food, altogether. There are no phases in the Ketogenic diet, like the Atkins. Keto allows the individual to start and maintain the weight loss by eating whole foods. Atkins has been criticized by the perception of shakes, bars, and freezer meals that a person needs in order to lose weight.

Keto has also been given credit to more than just weight-loss results. A number of studies result in Keto dieters having enhanced mental clarity and greater levels of energy. Keto is strict with macronutrients and steers a person to balance their macronutrients by eating whole, 'good fat' foods, unlike the Atkins diet. While the weight loss outcomes of the two diets may be similar, to begin with, the Atkins diet slowly reintroduces carbs to the body. This process makes it difficult for the body to maintain the initial weight loss that happens during the induction phase. Keto, however, relies on the same basis of macronutrients throughout the diet. That basis is high calories from fat (70%-80%), moderate calories from protein (20%-25%), and low calories from carbs (5%-10%). This same structure follows the dieter from beginning to end, thus projecting the significance of maintenance throughout the entire process.

The Atkins diet never differentiates on what types of foods can be consumed. It allows the dieter to consume processed foods, as long as it stays within the guidelines of the phase. For example, if you were to walk into a grocery store, you would find sections of aisles dedicated to the Atkins diet. Some of the items include pizzas, shakes, chocolate bars, and even candies. These items are simply low in net carbs (grams of carbs minus grams of fiber). They promote the use of bad ingredients like soy protein and certain sugar alcohols, which have links to other health problems. On the back of any given Atkins bar wrapper, you could also see the use of artificial sweeteners, which have been known to cause more problems than their rivals; natural sweeteners.

The overall goal of Keto is to rid the body of food toxins, which the Atkins diet doesn't address, but rather, promotes in some cases. The Atkins diet allows the consumer to go out and grab a highly processed pack of bacon, and grain-fed, processed meat. Keto emphasizes the consumption of grass-fed, organic meats as well as healthy fats. It strays away from all processed food and relies heavily on foods that are natural but have low levels of sugars, grains, and starches.

Hidden Benefits of the Ketogenic Diet

The benefits of the Ketogenic are vast. We've already discussed some of the benefits, but there are many more! Firstly, the diet increases memory, cognition as well as clarity. Researchers believe that the use of Ketones in place of glucose makes the brain recall events more clearly. Serious studies are being conducted in hopes of deterring early onsets of the Alzheimer's disease. The reason as to why people on the Keto diet have a better mental focus revolves around the idea that carbs as the main energy source give rise and fall to blood sugar levels in the body. This isn't consistent. Hence, it is harder for the brain to stay focused for longer periods of time. When the body switches into Ketosis, using Ketones at its main source of energy, it has a consistent reliance on them to fuel the body at all times. This makes a person focus for a longer period of time. The mind doesn't become clouded.

You also have a more consistent energy pattern. Instead of the energetic ups and downs that come with a high carb intake, your body naturally taps into its unused resources (your fat storage) and provides itself with an even flow of energy. As long as your body is, and stays, in Ketosis, there won't be spikes in your energy levels that are normally caused by increases in blood sugar levels.

The Keto diet is also said to aid in the prevention of some heart-related diseases. Once again, this is due, in part, to the mass reduction and increased stability of glucose levels in the body. Keto dieters have also seen better cholesterol profiles. You might think, a lot of fatty, greasy food is going into your body now, so your cholesterol levels have got to be out of control. A common misconception is that all cholesterol is bad. That is simply not the truth. Cholesterol is a substance made by our livers or comes from the consumption of animal-based products. Whether you consume foods high in cholesterol levels does not necessarily matter because it will always be produced in the liver. The reason the body still produces it is because it is a vital part of the brain and nervous system. Around 25% of a body's cholesterol is found in the brain. It is a building block for some of the connective tissues. Some studies show that people with lower cholesterol levels (below 200) still suffer from heart attacks and strokes. It's actually an overwhelming amount, too. Particularly, a study entitled, The Framingham Heart Study, shows that 40% of its participants that suffered from a heart attack had a cholesterol level below 200. The same study noted that a cholesterol level below 180 actually triples the likelihood of a heart attack or stroke. If a cholesterol level is low, it is a sign of malnutrition. So, a higher cholesterol level is not a bad thing to have, although you do not want it to get too high. You would want to maintain a healthy cholesterol level in your body. The Keto diet, if done correctly, can provide that balance.

Another great benefit of the Ketogenic diet is the decrease of inflammation. Inflammation is defined as the redness, swelling, pain, tenderness and disturbed function to an area of the body. A majority of processed foods break down into glucose. The reduction of glucose metabolism reawakened a protein in the body that suppressed the inflammatory genes. This, in turn, reduced the risks of inflammatory-based illnesses as well as pain.

In addition to these health benefits, the Keto diet also curbs risks of other health-related diseases, like diabetes. Type II diabetes often occurs in adults over the age of 45 who are overweight. With this type of diabetes, the body rejects insulin or simply does not produce enough of it. It may seem strange to suggest a high-fat diet to someone who has type II diabetes, but once Ketosis takes effect and is in sync with the body, it shows great benefits. If you suffer from diabetes, you may want to start the Ketogenic process under the close supervision of a health professional. The switch from using glucose as energy to using fat could be dangerous. Always make sure you test your blood sugar levels while you are on the Keto diet. Sufferers of type II diabetes, once on the diet, notice fewer symptoms. Some even feel the need for less medication. They recognize and adapt to higher insulin sensitivity as well as lower blood pressure levels.

Additionally, the Keto diet improves acne. The modern western diet contains a lot of sugar. Researchers conclude that diet is one of the biggest influences of the prevalence of acne, although it cannot be confirmed. People that eat more whole foods do not have to produce as much insulin as people that eat lots of processed foods. The more insulin the body has to produce, or the more insulin impacts other molecules, the more out of whack the skin becomes. Some of the insulin-impacted molecules create oily sebum. An oily sebum is a fancy term for the wax-like coating that covers pores of hair follicles. It then forms a microcomedone—a clogged skin pore. If the microcomedone is close to the skin, then the skin's pigment will be oxidized by the air, causing it to turn black. If the microcomedone occurs deep within a hair follicle, it will turn white. These are known as whiteheads and blackheads. The formation of these is an ideal place for bacteria to breed, thus inflammation occurs. We see spots of redness, tenderness, and some swelling. The less insulin that is used, the better the skin will be. And to use less insulin in the body means eating whole foods rather than processed foods.

There are many more benefits to the Keto diet. You will feel more alert and less fatigued, and there are a few studies that conclude you will sleep better. Some benefits are still being researched. There are undergoing scientific studies that link better quality of life to cancer patients. Not only that, but some go as far as saying that the diet could greatly impact cancer cells in the body by essentially "starving them" of the glucose they need to grow. While there are no guarantees as of yet, there are some doctors pushing cancer susceptible people, maybe someone that runs a risk of cancer through genetics, toward the Keto-lifestyle.

Chapter 2: Let's Get Started: Ketogenic Diet Food Lists for Women

When it comes to losing weight, it is often harder for women to drop the extra pounds than it is for men. There are particular reasons why, but in general, the female body takes longer to adjust to dietary and lifestyle changes. We will get into the particulars later on. There are specific foods that help kick-start a women's journey on the Keto diet. Women's studies researchers suggest adding more alkaline foods into the diet than recommended. Our bodies have a pH balance that helps us measure the acidity in our blood. If our blood becomes too acidic, it can affect our overall state of health. It is also an optimal place for the growth of illnesses—and even cancers.

The reason researchers push women to eat more alkaline foods is that they contain more nutrients. Foods that are highly acidic have little to no nutrients in them. They promote an array of problems that are meant to be corrected by the Keto diet. Some of those symptoms include:

- Low levels of energy
- Exhaustion
- Acne
- Clouded brain or confusion
- Anxiety
- Joint Pain
- Headaches
- Digestive problems like bloating

The Potential Renal Acid Load scale measures the acidity of a food by a positive, neutral, or negative value. The more negative numbers are the highest alkaline foods. This is not to be confused with the typical, more widely known pH scale. The pH scale is the opposite, which ranges from 0 to 14. The closer to zero, the more acidic a food is. The more alkaline foods are, the closer to 14 they are on the pH scale. Now, let's talk about what types of alkaline foods women could eat on Keto:

Spinach, which has a PRAL (Potential Renal Acid Load: How acidic or alkaline a food is once it's been metabolized) of -11.8. It's highly alkaline and dense in calcium.

Kale has a PRAL of -8.3. Once again, it is highly alkaline and is dense in calcium, iron, and Vitamin K.

Celery has a PRAL of -5.2. Celery is mostly water, which promotes cleansing properties. It can help flush toxins from the body.

Cauliflower has a PRAL of -4.0. Cauliflower is a great food source for Keto-dieting women. It has properties that can aid in balancing hormone levels when they are too high. High hormone levels can have a harmful effect on the body. It can also lead to weight gain, digestive problems like bloating, as well as infertility.

Eggplant has a PRAL of -3.4. Eggplant is also a great food source. It contains phytonutrients like chlorogenic acid. This is a plant compound that helps promote digestion and metabolism.

Zucchini has a PRAL of -2.6. It is a great source of the phytonutrient, lutein, which protects eyesight.

Broccoli has a PRAL of -4.0. It improves skin, metabolism, a healthy immune system and is anti-inflammatory. It also contains a lot of Vitamin K and Vitamin C.

Avocado has a PRAL of -8.2. This is considered the holy grail of Keto dieters. Avocado has a high healthy fat content. It speeds up metabolism and is an anti-inflammatory. It contains a high percentage of Vitamin K, Vitamin C, and potassium.

Bell Peppers have a PRAL of -3.4. They are a powerhouse for decreasing the risks of cardiovascular disease and type II diabetes. They also contain high amounts of Vitamin C, Vitamin A, Vitamin B6, and folate.

Another great food umbrella for women to eat from while on Keto is foods that are high in protein. Protein promotes the release of hormones, which can be a woman's pitfall on Keto, that control appetite. Ghrelin is a peptide hormone found primarily in the stomach. This particular hormone triggers the secretion of growth hormones from the pituitary gland and increases appetite. Eating more protein decreases the amount of ghrelin in the body. Moreover, it actually increases the hormones that help promote a feeling of fullness. A few foods that are high in protein and low in carbs are:

Fish, depending on what type you enjoy, contains a plethora of protein. Some examples of fish to eat that are high in protein and still Keto-friendly are salmon, which can contain upwards of 39 grams of protein per half of a fillet. Let's not forget about tuna. Tuna is a protein powerhouse. It can contain up to 43 grams of protein per half of a fillet.

Chicken is also a good source of protein. Depending on the size of a chicken breast, it can contain around 54 grams of protein per breast.

Eggs are another way to get the daily amount of protein into your diet. A single, large egg has 6 grams of protein.

Nuts also contain high levels of protein. Almonds contain around 20 grams of protein per cup. Pistachios are toward the top of the protein list, containing 25 grams per cup. Hazelnuts are also a great source, containing 20 grams of protein per cup.

Peanut Butter is also a moderate source of protein. Per 2 tbsp. of peanut butter (32 grams), there are 8 grams of protein.

Jerky is an easy way to get a source of protein. It can contain upwards of 9 grams per ounce of jerky (28 grams).

The good thing about foods such as peanut butter and nuts is that they are an easy on-the-go snack. They can easily be eaten by themselves. They can also be paired with other foods. Easy on-the-go, portable snacks can include:

- Peanut butter and celery

- Mixed nuts; trail mix not containing fruits or chocolate pieces
- Hard-boiled eggs
- Jerky sticks
- Cheese Slices
- Dippable veggies

These snacks and many more are great for a woman with a busy lifestyle that still wants to be a Keto dieter!

What Are Good Fats and Bad Fats?

The term good fats sound sort of oxymoronic but there is such a thing! To fully understand what a good fat is, we have to look at all types of fat and what makes them either good for you or bad.

There are three types of fat. Those include saturated, unsaturated, and trans fats. The most notable to avoid is trans fats. There are two types of trans fats found in food. Some of those, but not most, are naturally occurring trans-fat. Naturally occurring trans fats are produced inside an animal's gut and transfer into the foods of said animals. Some of the examples include some red meats and milk. The other type of trans fat is artificial. These types of fats are created by a process in which hydrogen is added to vegetable oils to make them more solid. It is also the most common of the two types of trans fats. The reason it is the most common is simple: it is cheap and easy to use. Trans fats raise the bad cholesterol in your body, which is also known as LDL cholesterol (low-density lipoprotein). This type of cholesterol is what most of us think of as the bad cholesterol in terms of the likelihood of having a heart attack or stroke. It acts as the plaque that clogs arteries.

The easiest way to get trans-fat into your system is by consuming fried and baked foods. Things like donuts, muffins, cookies, cakes, pie crusts, French fries, and biscuits contain trans-fat. The list goes on, but the main culprits can be found in your nearest drive-thru restaurant. You can tell if a product contains trans fats by reading the nutritional label located on most food packages. If a product contains less than .5 grams of trans fat, the producer is not required to label the product as containing it. Sort of scary, right?

Unsaturated fats are also broken down into two categories. The first is monounsaturated fats. This is where you get a lot of your healthy fats. These types of fats can help lower the bad (LDL) cholesterol in your body. Consuming more of the monounsaturated fats also helps lower the risk level of certain types of cardiovascular diseases. While it is not known, some researchers believe that this type of fat can also help control insulin levels and blood sugar. Monounsaturated fats can be found in avocados and avocado oil, olive oil, peanut oil, most nuts, and most seeds.

Polyunsaturated fats are needed in order for the body to function. While they are vital, it is difficult to say whether they are 'good fats' or 'bad fats'. This type of fat can be further divided into Omega-3 fatty acids and Omega-6 fatty acids. Omega-3 fatty acids can be found in fish, flaxseed oil, sunflower seeds, and walnuts. These types of fats are said to be good for the heart.

Omega-6 is debatable. Some believe it is good to help prevent cardiovascular diseases, but not enough is known to determine this as true. Researchers are also unsure of its role as an anti-inflammatory. Omega-6 fatty acids can be found in sunflower oil, soybean oil, and corn oil.

Finally, let's take a look at saturated fats. For years, saturated fats have been seen as harmful. They were said to have increased the risk of heart problems. More recent studies have debunked these myths. In fact, a specific type of saturated fat called medium-chain triglycerides (MCTs) are now known to be digested very easily. Things like coconut oil are MCTs. Once they are eaten, they are immediately passed to the liver and used for energy. They are a great tool to use for weight loss! Saturated fats are known to heighten levels of high-density lipoproteins (HDL). The body needs HDL, or good cholesterol, in order to remove LDL from the body. The more HDL cholesterol you have in your body, the less likely you are to suffer from heart-related diseases. HDL cholesterol acts as a janitor. It cleans the inner walls of your blood vessels, making them healthier. This is important because once the inner walls of your blood vessels become damaged, you are more susceptible to have a heart attack or stroke. While saturated fats increase your levels of HDL, they also take small, dense LDL and make them bigger and less dense, which is good. They do not affect the overall blood lipid profile like the previous thought.

Proteins to Enjoy and to Avoid

If you are looking to start the Ketogenic diet, there are certain foods to enjoy and to avoid. The next few sections will go into depth about what sorts of macronutrient-rich food you should eat. We've already touched on a few examples, but these sections will go deeper into what your diet could look like while on Keto. Variety is important, so let's get started.

Protein is a huge part of the Keto diet. It makes up between 20% and 25% of the foods you should eat. It is essential in the building of muscle and protecting it, regulation of hormones, tissue growth, and the immune system. Here are some proteins to enjoy while on the Keto diet:

- Seafood – most seafood are high in protein and contain very low amounts of carbs, if any.
  – Catfish, cod, flounder, tuna, salmon, trout, mackerel, mahi-mahi
- Some vegetables – some vegetables are low in carbs and high in protein. Steer away from vegetables that contain starches.
  – Cauliflower, broccoli, bell peppers, spinach, some mushrooms, eggplant, celery
- Cheese – there are hundreds of types of cheeses. Virtually all of them are low in carbs and high in protein. They are also good sources of fat!
- Meat and Poultry (grass-fed) – most meat and poultry are considered staples of the Keto diet. There are hardly carbs, if any, and they are also a rich source of protein.
  – beef, chicken, duck, lamb, pork, turkey, ham, deer
- Eggs – eggs are ideal for the Keto diet. They are less than one carb and have around 6 grams of protein.

- Greek Yogurt and Cottage Cheese – both of these items contain a higher number of carbs (around 5 grams) but are healthy and high in protein. They also create the feeling of being full.

Here are some proteins to avoid:
- Whey Protein – whey is a protein that comes from milk. It can also be formed as a byproduct of cheese-making. Whey is highly insulinogenic. Insulinogenic means of, relating to, or stimulating the production of insulin. The entire goal of the Ketogenic diet is to make insulin levels, as well as blood sugar levels, stable and low. Consuming whey disrupts the stability given to your insulin levels while in Ketosis. Some researchers believe consuming whey protein triggers an effect of insulin spikes much like the consumption of white bread.
- Tilapia – Surprisingly, tilapia, while it is a great source of protein, might not be as healthy as you might think. Its ratio of Omega-3 fatty acids to Omega-6 fatty acids concerns health professionals, for one. However, there are thoughts that tilapia also may lead to inflammation.

The Food and Drug Administration (FDA) has also released reports of concerning farming practices when it comes to tilapia. The United States gets most of its tilapia from China, where fish-farming practices include feeding fish other animal feces. This is not to say that tilapia is not a good source of protein, or not healthy because it is. But tilapia need very little nutrition to survive. China provides the United States with over 70% of its consumer-ready tilapia. Another report released by the FDA was said that over 187 shipments of tilapia contained harmful chemicals and pesticide additives. One of these additives is named Methyltestosterone. Methyltestosterone is essentially a steroid that aids the tilapia in its growth. While most countries have banned this additive, the United States still allows it.

- Too much protein – Consuming too much protein can actually kick your body out of Ketosis. If you eat an access to protein, it can actually raise your insulin levels. Your body will recycle the excess protein you do not need and turn it into glucose in a process called gluconeogenesis.

- Cold cuts of meat with added sugar – While some cold cuts of deli meat might be okay on this diet, you have to read labels. A number of deli meats contain additives such as sugar or corn starch. Sugar is what you want to avoid on this diet. Cornstarch is used as a thickening agent to plump up deli meats. It makes them last longer. Cornstarch is used as a replacement of flour in some recipes. Most measurements of cornstarch are cut in half when replacing the flour. So say a recipe contains one cup of flour, you would only use half a cup of cornstarch. Even then, half a cup of cornstarch is over 58 grams of net carbs with little to no dietary fiber to help you knock that number down. It would immediately knock you out of Ketosis. This isn't to say that deli meat is bad on the Keto diet, because they are a great source of protein, but watch the labels and read the nutritional facts before purchasing them.

- Protein is an essential part of this diet, but it is very important to still watch what you are putting into your body. Things such as whey protein, tilapia, and cold cuts of meat are just a few ways bad types of protein can make its way into your body. Also, you don't want to eat too much protein. Be mindful of what sorts of ingredients, rather than foods, you are eating and placing inside your body.

Carbs to Enjoy and to Avoid

A lot of foods we think of as healthy or healthier alternatives actually contain carbs. For example, we think of vegetables as generally healthy. Sure, they have a vast amount of nutrients. But they also contain a lot of carbs. And you want to avoid those as much as possible while doing Keto. It is impossible to avoid all carbs, which is why the Keto diet offers a set amount of carbs per day. The lower intake of carbs, the better off you will be and the faster you will get your body into Ketosis.

Here are some examples of carbs you should enjoy:

- Leafy vegetables – some vegetables are low in carbs. Steer away from vegetables that contain starches. A good rule of thumb is to stick to vegetables that are grown above the ground.
  – Cauliflower, broccoli, bell peppers, spinach, some mushrooms, eggplant, celery
- Nuts and Seeds – they are low in carbs, all-the-while contain high levels of fiber, nutrients, and fats.
  – Almonds, pistachios, hazelnuts, pecans, brazils, macadamia
- Berries – some of the fruits that you can consume while on the Keto diet are berries. They are lower in carbs than other fruits and they also add antioxidants to your diet. Be careful, though, an excessive number of berries can pile on carbs quickly.
  – Strawberries, raspberries, blackberries, blueberries (in moderation), plums
- Fiber Supplements – this is an indigestible carb that guides the digestive system into regulating blood glucose levels and immune system functionality.
  – Acacia, Psyllium Husk
- Avocados – This single food item needs to be categorized by itself. This fruit, while it may be higher in carbs than the previously listed foods, is a Keto staple. It is both high in fiber and high in fat. A single avocado can contain as little as 10 carbs but as much as 17 carbs per avocado. The good thing about this food is the net carbs. Because an avocado is high in fiber as well, it is lower in net carbs, all-the-while still containing upwards of as much as 22 grams of fat! It also contains vitamins such as zinc, iron, and magnesium. It is a great low net carb food.

Now, of course, with the good comes the bad. The 'bad' thing about these types of foods is they are potentially good for you but not on the Keto diet. Here are some bad carbs you'll want to avoid:

- **Grains such as wheat, rye, and corn.** These grains are things we have grown up with; things that we feel when we eat, we are being healthy. When it comes to Keto, this is the group of foods you want to keep away from.

– bread, pasta, cookies, cakes, pizza, buns
- **Legumes such as beans and soy.** They are good for you, in small quantities, for a nutrients supply. Legumes have been around forever, but there is a huge carb intake that comes with eating legumes. Eating a single cup of beans, for example, can have upwards as much as 40 carbs and only 15 grams of fiber. That still leaves you with 25 net carbs. And based on whichever Keto diet you are doing, or however many carbs you are allowed per day, this could be your entire serving!
– chickpeas, beans, peas, soy
- **Root vegetables such as carrots.** Root vegetables contain way more carbs than vegetables grown above ground. This does not mean these vegetables are 'bad' for you as they contain many nutrients. But they are definitely higher in the carb count. It is safer to avoid these types of vegetables.
– carrots, onions, parsnip, beetroots
- **Starchy vegetables such as potatoes.** Once again, these vegetables are not 'bad'. They are simply higher in carbs than leafy green vegetables.
– potatoes, corn, squash, pumpkin, yams, sweet potatoes, plantain
- **Fruits such as apples.** These types of fruits are not only higher in carbs, but they also contain sugar. Sugar can cause spikes in insulin in the body. It is easier just to avoid high sugary fruits.
– apples, mangos, bananas, watermelon, peaches, oranges

These lists have a lot of foods listed on them, but it is not all of the foods you can eat on the Keto diet. There are plenty of low carb options to choose from. On Keto, variety is important.

Snacks to Enjoy

The Keto diet is one of the most satisfying diets for women. The types of foods that are consumed are relatively filling. Because of the regulations of hormones, blood sugar, insulin and ghrelin it is less likely to become hungry in between meals. That is not to say that it will not happen because it can. It is just less likely. There are a number of high fat, low carb, high protein snack options. Here are some of them:

High-Fat Snacks:
- Avocados – Are you tired of hearing about them, yet?
- Olives
- Pork rinds – These are a good alternative to crackers or chips if you are in that, 'can't just have one' mindset.
- Macadamia nuts
- Dark chocolate – Yes, you can have a Keto-friendly chocolate. It's hard to avoid chocolate, especially when you have cravings. Just make sure this snack has 80% or more cocoa content. The carbs could add up rather quickly.
- Pepperoni slices – Although they are super high in fat, they are highly processed so eat them sparingly.
- High-fat cheeses
- Peanut butter

High-Protein Snacks:
- Sardines
- Beef Jerky
- Cheese chips – a few brands actually make cheese chips. They are crispy chips made out of cheese rather than flour, like a cracker.
- Veggie sticks, like celery
- Hard-boiled eggs

More Low-Carb Snacks:
- Cherry tomatoes – You have to be mindful of how many tomatoes you eat because they do have some carbs.
- Keto chips – They do have added sugars, so you have to be mindful of how many you are eating.
- Guacamole
- Fat Bombs – Fat bombs are quick and easy snacks you can make at home.
- Deli meat and cheese wraps – Once again, be careful when selecting your deli meats.

- Nut butter
- Bone Broth
- Bulletproof coffee
- Sunflower seeds
- Cottage cheese – in moderation
- Pumpkin seeds
- Pickles
- Meatballs
- Avocado fries

There are different variations of some of these foods. For example, you can make meatballs a number of different ways. The same goes for things like avocado fries, guacamole, and bulletproof coffee. And this is, by all means, not a complete list of all Keto-safe snacks. This is just a starting point in your Keto journey. There are also different types of foods called 'fat-bombs.'

Fat bombs have been popularized in the last few years. These are small round shaped snacks, usually sweet in nature, that have a high concentration of fat. Some of the ingredients include peanut butter, dark chocolate, nuts, and nut butter. And yes, avocados! They help keep you full while waiting on your next meal. If you are afraid you are not going to meet your total fat goal for the day, make a fat-bomb!

Common misconceptions about what things to drink on Keto are vast. One of the biggest pitfalls is drinking diet soda. Regular soda has been criticized among health professionals for years. It is packed with sugar. So, a lot of people believe that switching to diet soda is better. Sure, it has no carbs, no sugar, and tastes pretty similar to regular soda. But researchers believe that diet soda is actually worse for you than regular soda. It is packed with artificial ingredients, including sweeteners. It contains no protein and no fat and is high in sodium. When you consume a diet soda, the body senses a sweet sensation. It expects to receive high blood sugar and insulin, but it never happens. If you consume a lot of diet soda, these constant mixed signals could trigger a metabolic syndrome or type II diabetes.

A great drink alternative to avoid as much soda as possible is Mio. Mio does contain artificial sweeteners and artificial color as well, but all have been approved as safe by the Federal Drug Administration (FDA) as long as it is in small doses. Mio also provides different types of nutritional value. Some types of Mio have vitamins such as B3. B3 is also known as Niacin. Niacin is known to help treat type I diabetes. It is an essential part of our diet. It's also water-soluble so it doesn't get stored in the body. It is a great source of electrolytes as well. Some believe that Gatorade Zero is an option on Keto. The nutritional level of Gatorade is a bit high, though. A normal bottle of Gatorade has about 35 grams of carbs. A G2 version still contains about 12 grams. And the amount of sugar is a bit much. It can contain upwards of twelve grams of sugar. It is important to read the nutritional labels on such drinks to make sure your body isn't ingesting sugar and carbs that you do not want there. It could knock your body out of Ketosis.

Alcohol on Keto is another big restriction. It is best to use pure forms of alcohol to stay within Ketosis. Things such as gin, rum, vodka, tequila, and whiskey all contain zero carbs. But watch what you mix them with. Or you could drink them straight. Red wines and light beers are also okay. But light beers can pile on the carbs rather quickly. They can each contain upwards of 3-4 carbs per serving. Alcohol is also full of empty calories, which can make you hungry. The body treats alcohol as a toxin, too. So, it may slow down the fat burning process. Your body shifts focus from burning fat to pushing the toxins out of your body. Also, you may notice that you get drunker faster. The alcohol hits your system faster and stronger than it did before when your body wasn't in Ketosis. Typically, with a high carb diet, the body had a glycogen cushion built in to slow the metabolizing of alcohol. Without this cushion, the body has no buffer. So, it is best to limit the amount of alcohol you consume while on the Keto diet.

Essential Ketogenic Diet Guidelines for Women

Females typically have more of a body fat percentage than males. Most of that fat storage difference is because of pregnancies and how the woman's body adapts during adolescence. Women usually have between six and eleven percent more body fat than men.

Most of the fat deposits in a sex-related fashion and revolves around the hips, thighs, pelvis, and buttocks of a woman. After adolescence, fat cells do not typically multiply—rather, they grow. Researchers have noted that it is harder for women to lose weight when first starting on a diet, but usually, the weight loss evens out after about six months. It's hard to stay committed to a diet that doesn't give you fast results. Luckily with the Keto diet, you start seeing results within the first week. That makes this diet easier to stick to.

With this diet, there are guidelines for women to follow. Most of these guidelines are customizable. You have to find what works for you. But because our bodies are, more or less, the same when it comes to fattier tissue and deposit areas, here are some of the guidelines that might work for you!

First and foremost, the change will not happen overnight! You have to give yourself time. Drastically changing your eating habits is hard. Some women on Keto have told their stories, and they are too busy to eat low carb, high fat all the time. They can't go to the grocery store; they have to cook dinner for their families. And let's face it, no one wants to cook two different meals—one for you and one for your family. It's hard, but if this diet is for you, don't be hard on yourself to start because it does get easier. The internet has many different guides to help women when first starting a diet. Some sites also give out beginners shopping lists. Use your tools and realize you are not alone if the Keto diet starts off difficult for you. You mustn't get into a failure mindset, though. There is support!

Next, it is important to listen to your body. A hormone imbalance, for women, can really throw a wrench in your Keto plans. Do you crave sugars before your period? What about salt? Do you have severe PMS? Do you have problems focusing? Is your sex drive low? All of these things could be linked to what is called Adrenal Fatigue. While it is not used as a medical diagnosis, it can explain a lot of what you are feeling. Adrenal Fatigue is thought to be caused by chronic stress. Your body is too busy producing flight-or-fight arousal that it cannot produce enough hormones to feel good. Alternative medicine professionals believe this is a real diagnosis, but current blood testing cannot determine a root cause for Adrenal Fatigue. You may not take this at face value, but the symptoms still exist. This hormone imbalance could trigger a number of different things, like more stress! The adrenal gland is responsible for a high production of estrogen, especially in menopausal or pre-menopausal women. It is also responsible for the production of your stress hormones like adrenaline and cortisol. Cortisol is like your body's built-in alarm system. It is your body's main stress hormone. It works hand in hand with your brain to help keep you motivated and control your mood. If your body produces too much cortisol, because you are under a lot of stress or maybe you're not eating enough, it can throw your other hormones out of whack. Whacky hormones can lead to fatigue, weight gain, and irritability. If you ever feel like you could sleep all day, this could be the underlying problem. Your body is tired. During this period of fatigue or any period of fatigue, your body and brain give up. They cannot keep up with the amounts of stress in your world. Stress can, in turn, blow your body out of Ketosis. Higher levels of cortisol actually increase amounts of insulin in the body. The whole goal of the Keto diet is to lower levels of insulin, as well as many other things. If your insulin levels are lower, you actually lower the amounts of cortisol in your body. Your body then becomes less stressed and balances more of your hormones.

Once you develop your plan on Keto, try to stick to it. The key word here is trying! The most important part of this diet is that your body feels good and safe. If you are full at the end of the day, but you didn't eat enough fat or maybe you are low on protein, it is okay. If you are starving, eat—even if it isn't a part of your plan. Not eating can lead to some infertility issues. The more stress placed on your body, the less healed and nourished it is. This, in turn, sends messages to your body telling it is not ready to carry a child. It is thinking fight-or-flight and that there aren't enough calories to have a child. Your body will fight against you to become pregnant, telling you it isn't safe to have a baby. If your body is in starvation mode, it won't produce hormones.

A part of the Keto diet is intermittent fasting. This is where you cycle between periods of eating and not eating. Most Keto dieters fast while they sleep. If you sleep 8 hours every night, you are fasting without even thinking about it. Some people skip breakfast on their days to fast. Maybe they'll eat their first meal around noon. If you go to bed at midnight, you are fasting for 12 hours. The other part of intermittent fasting is the eating window. Once you have fasted, limit your time to eat in a block of time. If you eat your first meal at noon, maybe your next meal is at eight at night. So, you're eating block is between noon and eight while you are fasting. Hunger is not usually a problem while fasting because your body becomes accustomed to your eating patterns. This isn't to say it might not be a bit more difficult to start, but it will get easier. Some women have had success with drinking bullet-proof coffee, or tea while they are in their fasting stage as long as there are no/low amounts of carbs. There are still high amounts of fat in bullet-proof coffee (and some protein) so while fasting, it sends the message to your body that you are okay, and it shouldn't go into starvation mode. It also sends the message to your adrenal glands that you are safe.

Another key thing for women is to not completely cut yourself off from all carbs. The state of Ketosis is reached differently for everyone. It is more difficult for women because our hormones become chaotic with dietary change. To start the Keto diet, you may want to gradually cut back carbs. This could take two to four weeks, sometimes even more time, depending on how your body reacts. So, every once in a while, ask yourself how you feel. Are you still tired? Are you feeling hungry all of the time? If so, gradually add some carbs back into your diet, and then cut them back down again. You don't want your body to stress, because it creates more cortisol. The more cortisol in your body, the more insulin is produced.

Lastly, you have to know the best time to weigh yourself. The absolute best guideline is to keep it consistent. If you weigh yourself once a week, keep it on the same day at the same time, every time. Most Keto dieters weigh in the morning before eating. If your weight fluctuates a bit, it is hard not to get discouraged. But fear not! If your body is still in Ketosis, it is still fat-burning. The weight differences are usually from the large amounts of water that are needed in this diet.

These guidelines are meant to help. Being a woman on the Keto diet is difficult. There are many things women have to take into consideration that do not mean as much to men. Please remember,

30

these guidelines differ from person to person. And there are many more!

Common Mistakes on the Keto Diet and How to Overcome Them

There are quite a few common mistakes made on the Keto diet. It's hard! You are not only changing your diet; you are changing your lifestyle. It takes a lot of focus and a lot of drive to become fully Ketogenic. Your body is making a change, so you have to follow suit.

Here are some common mistakes that are made on the Keto diet and how you overcome them.

The first is not paying attention to how you feel. There is already some information listed above about this subject, but it's a big enough mistake and needs to be hit hard. A lot of people get caught up in whether or not they are losing weight. What matters is that you are being healthy. This isn't as simple as it may sound. But the truth with this diet is that if you are following guidelines, and you feel good about what you are putting into your body, the initial weight loss will follow.

Secondly, thinking it is all about the food you are putting into your body is a mistake. This sort of diet is a lifestyle change. Of course, you can make healthier eating choices, and you should. Along with the diet portion comes typical weight loss protocols. Exercising is very important. It helps boost along your weight loss journey. Physical activities also reduce the further risks of type II diabetes, cancers, and cardiovascular disease. Increasing the number of physical activities, you do per day also improves your quality of life. So, if you are a victim of the first mistake of not paying attention to how you are feeling, there is a remedy that could potentially help. Exercise can also help you sleep better, lower blood pressure levels, lower levels of bad cholesterol and build stronger muscles and bones.

Thirdly, do not try to force things to happen. Some things work for some people. Not everything that is in this audiobook will work for you. If intermittent fasting isn't up your alley, you do not have to do it. The goal here is to make you feel comfortable with doing Keto, all-the-while eating better and making healthier choices. If something isn't for you, it doesn't mean you can't be on the Keto diet. Sculpt this diet to fit your needs.

The biggest and the most important mistake is being afraid to make mistakes and comparing yourself to others. No two single people are the same or are built the same way. This is especially hard for women. There seems to be a standard that all women have to meet in order to be considered beautiful. While things are changing in the entertainment industry, it is still hard to not compare yourself to someone who is thinner, leaner, or more muscular. You have to do what is best for you. The only comparison to be made is to your previous self. Are you making improvements? Do you feel better about yourself? Are you happier? Are you healthier?

While it is important to consult with medical professionals and listen to what they have to say, it gets hard to determine what to do on this diet. You'll come to find out that doctors, Keto-bloggers, or research students do not agree on most things. If one doctor says to eat more greenery, and another says to eat more meat, what do you do? Try both! See what works best for you and stick to it! You have to do what is best for you and your body. You don't have to pick a side or stance. You can do whatever fits within your life. You can even switch it up after a while and change your mind. Keep all doors and options open with this diet.

Another mistake that is made on Keto, quite frequently, is snacking. Some people think that because there are no calorie restrictions, that they can eat as much as they want. This isn't necessarily true. Snacking can get out of hand rather quickly. Once you are on the diet, find a meal plan that works for you. Find foods that will keep you full longer. A high number of people on Keto don't feel like they need snacks because of how fulfilling their meals are. This may not be true for everyone. But this does not mean you should sit on the couch and eat pork rinds all day. Those calories add up, and simply put—it isn't good for you. A way to avoid this is to plan out a snack. Once you've gotten used to how your body feels on Keto, determine the best time to eat a snack during your day (a time you know you'll be hungry) and eat it. This suppresses the urge to go to your fridge every hour and eat a cheese stick or eat a spoonful of peanut butter.

Another common mistake is constantly striving for perfection. You are going to wear yourself down by trying to hit your macros every day. It is okay to be out of tune every once in a while, as long as you plan to correct it the next day. Being perfect is not sustainable. You might find yourself fasting only three or four days a week, or maybe only hitting your macros three days out of the week and that is okay. If you constantly stress about hitting your goals each and every day, chances are you will burn yourself out. Not to mention, stress could knock your body out of Ketosis. Just do what you feel you can do. If you can only change smaller things to start with, that is good! It is better than what you were doing. And if you feel like it, gradually add more changes to your lifestyle.

Another major mistake people make is falling into a uniformity of foods you can eat. Being on the Keto diet still allows for varieties of foods. You'll want to expand that variety to gain as much and as many nutrients as you can. The cool thing about Keto is if you think of a food that you really want, chances are, there is a Keto version of it. The internet is endless with recipes for Keto dishes and is a great resource to find something new and inventive to eat.

It is very common to not hold yourself accountable. That goes with any diet. Accountability goes a lot further than accepting responsibility for your actions. It is being able to justify why you did something. The thing about not working out for a couple of weeks or eating a cookie every once in a while is that it turns into a habit. While you are on this diet, ask yourself if it is worth it? You have to be honest with yourself. It might be a bit easier if you have been on this diet for a while because the food isn't used for entertainment anymore. It becomes something you need rather than want. If it helps, connect with other people who can support you on your journey. Do have those people who help you hold you accountable. You could join a group on a social media platform. You could do diet bets. Maybe you and a friend, or you and your spouse start this journey together. See who can out-diet who.

Another mistake is not measuring your macros at all. In order to be successful on this diet, you have to know what you are putting into your body. There are numerous apps that you can download to keep track of your macros. Once you have been accustomed to certain foods and how much you can eat, maybe measuring macros isn't right for you. But in order to begin, it is important to know what sorts of foods help you hit your goals.

The last mistake to mention is one that is all too common and is probably the hardest to correct. You simply aren't eating enough fat. Most people have a fat-phobia, meaning they feel like putting too much fat into your body can clog arteries and cause heart attacks. This isn't true. This myth has been dispelled since the 50s. This high-fat diet is just that: high in fat. You have to consume enough fat to make up for the loss of carbs. If this doesn't happen, you could plateau. The same goes with not having enough protein in your diet. This means that after the initial drop in weight, you could go months without losing any more. There is a chance that your macros aren't where they need to be. You have to eat fat! And lots of it!

There are a number of trial and tribulations you need to overcome while on the Keto diet. Listen to what your body is telling you and work with it, not against it. These common mistakes could be costing you a lot more than what you think. But, where this is a will, there is a way. Don't get discouraged if you have been doing some of these things. It's okay. Move forward!

Chapter 3: Tips to Adapt to the Ketogenic Lifestyle

Common Pitfalls Women Face on the Ketogenic Diet and How to Overcome Them

The Ketogenic diet is different for women than it is for men. One of the main reasons is something we have already discussed—hormones. Women are more sensitive when it comes to hormones. We have a cycle that our bodies go through, and being on the Keto diet acts as a healer. Once again, you can't just drop everything that you are eating today and start off with no/low carbs tomorrow. It is a process, and a woman's body is delicate. It takes time to switch a diet and have your body follow up with you to know how you are doing—and the results all depend on how you feel. If you feel healthier, more awake, less fatigued, and less clouded, you are doing something right for yourself.

Some women, once transitioning to the Keto diet, don't get enough electrolytes. That is because there is not as much sodium and potassium in whole foods as there is in processed foods. So once you make the switch, make sure that you find a way to get electrolytes into your system. Not having enough electrolytes in your system can result in a few different problems. One would be cravings. Your body is so used to the amount of sodium, that it craves it once it's not getting any. Cravings are hard to deal with because it can be a "reason to live" so to speak. This means that it controls you, and it is literally all you can think about. Make sure you load up on foods that are high in potassium and sodium. Avocados and spinach are great sources!

When women think about the Keto diet, they begin thinking about the amount of fat they have to eat. When you are basing a high-fat diet solely on fat, you probably aren't getting enough of the nutrient-dense, leafy greens. This is hard because a lot of people know veggies are high in carbs, so they tend to think they should just avoid them altogether. This is not the case. Things such as kale, broccoli, and spinach are essential to this diet to get adequate nutrition into your body.

When you get on the Keto diet, exercise is very important alongside the foods you will be eating. Exercising actually drains your glycogen storage. This is where glucose is stored in the body. Thus, the more you exercise, the easier it is and the faster you get into Ketosis. Always find a way to do a bit of exercise in your daily routine. It could be as simple as taking a short walk with your dog. Try to exercise for around thirty minutes per day.

Another pitfall of women on the Keto diet is forcing the body to fast. In short, if you are hungry, eat. If you are full, stop eating. While the percentages of macros in your diet are important, you have to listen to your body. Don't fast for the sake of fasting. You have to do what is genuinely best for you.

A lot of these problems and mistakes can actually make women last longer in what is called the Keto-flu. There will be more discussion on that later on. It is just important to balance your new lifestyle. Rather than just eating the right types of foods, you have to exercise, replenish key electrolytes, and make sure you are doing only what you need to do—not what everyone else *thinks* you should do.

Does the Ketogenic Diet Suit You?

The short answer to this question is yes. In some form, the Keto diet is a great way to eat and be healthy. Let's go a little more in depth. There are four types of Ketogenic diets, so there are a lot more options for you if the standard Ketogenic diet (SKD) does not work for you.

The second type is called the cyclical Ketogenic diet (CKD). This sort of diet involves two days of heavy carb eating and then five days of the standard Keto diet. If you are super athletic or work out a lot, this may be the type of Keto diet for you. The two days of high carb loading helps refill muscles in order to retain them during rigorous work out periods.

The third type of Keto diet is called the targeted Ketogenic diet. This diet allows you to add carbs just around work out times. It's like a mixture of the SKD and CKD. This allows you to still get the carbs you need in order to retain muscle during workouts, but you are not out of Ketosis for days at a time. It is just short periods of time during the day. If you do moderate workouts and aren't involved in any strength training, then the SKD is what you need.

The last type of Keto diet is called the high-protein Ketogenic diet. This is similar to SKD but overall, it has more proteins and less fat. The ratio often looks like this: 60% fats, 35% proteins, and 5% carbs. This is ideal for people who are looking to build muscle mass or slow the breakdown of it. Most people who are on this diet are bodybuilders and older people. It is also good for people who show signs of protein deficiency. If you have a protein deficiency, it can show by the loss of muscle mass or by thinning hair.

Pick which diet is best for you. Professionals warn about the process of Keto-cycling, though while on the CKD. Keto-cycling is the process of eating carbs and then restricting yourself again. It can be dangerous to the body in terms of fluctuations of body water. These changes can lead to dizziness and can potentially worsen heart conditions. Always consult with your doctor before beginning a diet and determine which one is right for you.

If you are busy and are having problems trying to figure out if the Ketogenic diet best suits you and your life, the chances are it couldn't hurt. If you are looking to increase your overall wellbeing, it is suited for you. If you are looking to lose weight, it is suited for you. If you would like to introduce more nutrients into your diet, it is suited for you. The good thing about the Keto diet is that it could be integrated into any lifestyle. If you feel as if you are too busy to adapt to these changes, no worries. There is no rush. You can slowly integrate this diet into your life. It is actually recommended that you gradually change your eating habits over a two to four-week period.

If you are afraid of being a woman of convenience, there's nothing to fear. It is ten times easier to go through a drive-thru or order a pizza for dinner rather than cooking. But a lot of fast-food places offer Keto-friendly foods. You just have to research what you can eat from these places of ease. The Keto diet adapts to many different types of lifestyles. Find one that works for you.

The Lack of Fiber

Some people fear that with the decrease in carbs on the Keto diet, it will be difficult to get enough fiber into their body. You have to cut out the majority of fruits and all starchy vegetables, so how do you get fiber into your diet? The term dietary fiber refers to the indigestible part of the plant food that travels through our digestive system. Fiber helps prevent constipation as well as protects against heart disease, gastrointestinal health, maintains healthy insulin levels for diabetics, and aids in weight loss.

There are two types of fiber. The first one is soluble fiber. This type of fiber binds together with fatty acids in the body. It is very important to make sure you are eating the right types of foods for this fiber to be prominent in the body. It has a very important function. After it binds to the fatty acids, it slows them down which, in turn, takes them longer to empty out of the stomach. Therefore, you feel fuller for longer periods of time. Furthermore, it also slows down the rate at which the body absorbs sugar. Soluble fiber lowers bad LDL and regulates sugar intake as a whole. This is helpful for people that are diabetic. Some foods that will help you increase your soluble fiber levels are flaxseeds, chia seeds, coconut, spinach, and avocado.

The second type of fiber is insoluble fiber. It helps move solid waste through the digestive tract. It also helps control pH levels in the intestines. This type of fiber has a number of benefits, also. Insoluble fibers speed up the waste removal process of the body. It also promotes regular bowel movements and prevents constipation. Some foods that will help you increase your insoluble fiber levels are cauliflower, raspberries, and broccoli.

Soluble fiber dissolves in water whereas insoluble does not. Insoluble fiber actually never changes its shape as it travels through the digestive system. Soluble fiber does change but never completely breaks down. As it absorbs water, it becomes more gelatinous. Insoluble is stronger and does not break down as it pushes through your digestive tract. Some people think of it as a scouring pad moving through your body. It pushes things where they need to go and cleans up any mess left behind. Soluble fiber makes it harder for your body to break down carbs and process them into glucose. In turn, this lowers the intensity of blood sugar spikes in your body which then, regulates insulin levels.

If your intake of fiber is low, it is hard to satisfy that feeling of being full. Ultimately, because you are snacking more often to feel satisfied, you can potentially reverse your weight loss progress on Keto. It can even knock your body out of Ketosis.

If you have a good amount of fiber in your diet, you can usually tell by not feeling constipated. This differs from person to person. The same amount of dietary fiber is not going to be the same for everyone. So, find a level of fiber that works best with your body. Another important rule of thumb is to drink plenty of water while on Keto. There is a more likely chance that you could become dehydrated as the fiber in your body is absorbing and holding on to water.

Fiber is very important while on the Keto diet. But there are things to watch out for. One of those things is called isomaltooligosaccharides (IMO). IMOs can be made in a few different ways. They are all mostly derived from a sugar called maltose. IMOs are promoted as a dietary fiber with a hint of sweetness. They are predominantly found in nutrition bars, healthy cookies, and candies. The problem with them is that they are promoted as fibers, but do not break down the same way. Once they start breaking down, IMOs can actually turn into glucose and maltose. Because they have to potential to create high blood glucose levels, they could also create spikes in insulin which is what Keto dieters are trying to avoid.

So, what do you need to know about fiber and carbs? When you look at food labeling and notice the term net carbs, it means the total number of carbs minus grams of fiber. For example, if you are consuming a protein bar and it says it has 4 net carbs, but you turn it over and it reads 25 carbs, that means there are 21 grams of fiber in that item. That gives you your total net carbs. Net carbs are tricky though. Before you begin the Keto diet, ask yourself about your goals and what you want to get out of being on this diet. If you are more sensitive to the carb take away that occurs on the diet, maybe measuring net carbs is better for you. Some people who, rather than lose weight, want to maintain it measure their carb intake by using net carbs. Others who may want to lose more measure total carbs. It is up to you, your body and what you can handle. It may even switch for you while on the diet. Instead of measuring total carbs, you switch to measuring net carbs and vice versa.

A lot of dieters forget about fiber, which is why they run into digestive problems like constipation. People get caught up in the low carb, high-fat part of the diet too easily. Always remember your fiber because it can also aid in weight loss. Fiber is a tool that can change and affect bacteria in your gut. The change in bacteria can change the ability to burn fat. There was a specific study done in Canada to confirm this. Doctors took a group of kids who were obese. Half of the kids received extra fiber in their diet for sixteen weeks; the other group did not receive the added fiber. What doctors learned is that the group of children's, who received the extra fiber, body composition completely changed. Their gut microbiomes also changed. Those children lost 2.4% more body fat than the children that did not receive fiber. The take away here is simply not to forget about fiber and your leafy green vegetables. Yes, you need to increase fat intake. Yes, you need to lower your carb intake, but it is important not to do so at the expense of your fiber consumption. Fiber is your friend.

Too Much Protein

Consuming too much protein can be damaging to your body. If you are using protein as a way to lose weight, it can actually make you gain weight in the long haul. That is why it is so important to count your macros. A set amount of protein is essential to almost all diets. It helps repair and strengthen the muscle. It even creates new muscle. It also helps build strong bones, organs, and maintains healthy brain function.

Protein is essential on the Ketogenic diet. There is a process the body goes through while in Ketosis. First and foremost, the body will always, always go for glucose to burn for energy if it is in the body. That is why you minimize the number of carbs eaten in a day. If the body can't get to the glucose that it needs, it will go for muscle protein and break it down in a process called *gluconeogenesis,* which means making new sugar. This is why it is so important to eat enough protein. If you eat a certain amount of protein a day, the body will defer from using muscle protein and resort to using the protein you've eaten in your foods to create new sugar. This entire process is being aided by the fat you are consuming. When the fat burns, the liver releases Ketones and provides the energy to conduct this activity in your body.

How do you know the correct amount of protein to eat in a day? There is a good equation to go by, and that some medical professionals actually recommend. For every pound that you weigh, you would need between .3 grams and .7 grams of protein. So, for example, say you weigh 200 pounds. You would take 200 and multiply it by .3 or whatever amount of protein you think you need. That equals 60 grams of protein per day. You would need more protein (.7 grams) if you worked out regularly.

A regular, consistent source of protein is recommended on the Keto diet. Configure how much protein you need in a single day and find good sources through Keto-approved foods. There is a wide variety of foods and resources to pick from, just be careful not to overdo it. Too much protein can affect your kidneys and cause kidney stones. It can also strain your liver. Make sure you are careful when counting grams of protein. When you are consuming .7 grams per pound of weight, it can become excessive, especially when you are not working out on a regular basis. Excessive protein will also create more fat in your body. The proteins that are not needed to carry out certain functions of the body are converted to sugar.

Protein affects the body differently for women, as well. Women's bodies are on a monthly cycle. Depending on which point you are at on your cycle, proteins can affect Ketone levels differently. During the luteal phase, for example, women are more likely to consume protein and have it not affect their Ketone levels. During a follicular phase, however, that exact amount of protein may decrease

Ketone production. One of the easiest ways to find a personal protein limit is to purchase a Blood-Ketone meter. These are commonly used by people with diabetes and Keto-dieters. The meter does read differently for people on Keto. A normal Ketogenic state will have a reading between 0.5 and 3 mmol/L. It may take some time to get these results but stick with it! At certain points, it may read differently, and that is okay. It all depends on where you are at in your monthly cycle. Eventually, you will get an understanding of when your Ketone levels are good and when they drop a bit—if they do at all. Retaining an adequate amount of protein in your diet and in your body can help you to stay regular.

Dehydration

Your body is over 50% water. When starting a low carb diet, your body experiences loss of water. This is more likely to happen at the beginning of the diet when your body goes through a rapid change it is not used it. So, always be mindful of how much water you need in your diet.

If you feel dehydrated when first starting on Keto, here is why! Whenever you consume a carb, it is stored in the form of glycogen. Glycogen is a polysaccharide (a carbohydrate that has molecules of sugar bonded together) that forms glucose. From there the body automatically stores three to four grams of water. It does so because of glucose spikes levels of insulin in the body. When there is a spike of insulin in the body, the kidneys tell the rest of the body to hold onto water. When you are on a low carb diet, that process does not occur. The kidneys stop sending the signal to the rest of the body. They don't need to hold on to as much water as they did before. So, they tell the body it is okay to get rid of the excess water. This is why people feel better within days of starting the Keto diet. Because you are getting rid of the excess water in your body, inflammation also goes down. There's a reduction in edema. Edema is the medical term for swelling. This is usually caused by sodium. Sodium creates the ability to hold on to that water. On the diet, you are not consuming as much sodium as you used to, so it is easy to see results within days. You may even see a couple of pounds missing from the scale.

Because the kidneys are no longer sending the signal to the rest of the body to retain water, you may find yourself peeing more often. This is a good sign that you are headed in the right direction but it can also go too far. When you urinate, you are not only losing water, you are also losing sodium. Sodium, in this case, is not your average table salt. Sodium is very important for proper bodily function as it contains a lot of minerals. The problem people run into is not being able to replenish the lost sodium. Low carb foods don't have a lot of good sodium in them. So, what happens is that you lose all of the good sodium minerals and replace them with bad sodium minerals. Once this happens, dieters begin losing other minerals like potassium and magnesium. Then you are left with a bad mineral balance. With that, we lose the ability to function on all cylinders. Our nerves do not fire in the proper way. This causes you to feel weak. Your electrolytes are depleted. When you feel weak, your appetite is not there. When your appetite is not there it is harder to drink water.

So how do you overcome dehydration and replenish your body? The first thing is to add some sodium back into your body. This can be done by using Himalayan pink salt or Hawaiian black sand sea salt, or basically any type of sea salt—just not iodized table salt. The first step into rehydrating your body is to increase your sodium. At this point in time, your intake needs to be a little bit higher than normal. Most researchers suggest 3-5 grams of sodium to start off. This will help correct the sudden mineral imbalance your body just went through. If you plan on working out one day, make sure you increase the amounts of sodium before you do so. Once you start sweating, you are depleting your sodium stores. Remember, your kidneys aren't working like they used to. If you don't replenish before you begin your workout, you will resort back to being weaker once you're done, so always eat more sodium before a workout and not after. Plus, the increase in sodium before gives you the energy boost you may need to make it through.

Also, to stay hydrated there is a key thing that you could do. It is drink water. Water is super important while you are on a low carb diet, for the reasons listed above. Dehydration can cause many symptoms that can throw your body out of whack. Some of them are:

- Less frequent urination
- Dizziness
- Confusion
- Fatigue
- Extreme thirst
- Dark-colored urine
- Bad breath
- Constipation
- Dry skin
- Headaches

If you experience any of these symptoms, you may be dehydrated. If you can't get to a source of water and you start to feel any of these symptoms, caffeine is a good source, regardless of what some researchers might say. Caffeine makes you have to urinate, meaning it gives the signs that you may become dehydrated quickly. This isn't the case. There are properties of caffeinated beverages that offset the loss of fluid in the body. This isn't the only way to become hydrated quickly, though. Here some ideas on how to hydrate quickly.

- Eat something salty
- Eat raspberries or blueberries
- Lie down (conserve energy)
- Eat broth
- Eat Greek yogurt
- Drink fresh coconut water
- Green smoothies
- Eat water-rich vegetables

Make sure to listen to your body and watch for signs of dehydration, especially while your body is going into Ketosis. It's hard to determine if your body is dehydrated, but hopefully, these tips help out. This is not a complete list of what dehydration looks like or feels like, but it could give you a sign while you are on the Keto diet.

What is the Ketogenic Flu, and How to Get Over It?

If you are starting to research the Ketogenic diet, you might come across terms such as 'Keto sickness,' or 'Keto virus.' These are all referring to the most common use of its name, the Keto flu. There are many symptoms associated with the Keto flu. They much resemble influenza. But there are reasons why your body is acting like it is sick. And truthfully, it is but you are working toward a healing process.

The first reason your body is acting like it's sick is that you are going through a withdraw. Eating carbs, sugars, and things alike triggers the reward system in the brain. Having those things in your system releases dopamine. Dopamine is a neurotransmitter responsible for sending messages from your nerve cells to your brain. When your body doesn't receive the sugar and carbs that it is used to, those messages are not sent. Your body has a negative response. Sometimes, it goes as far as being depressed and getting irritable.

Another part of the Keto flu is best explained using an example. When you are burning through the last of the carbs in your body, you feel okay. But you haven't tapped into the best source yet. Think of your gas tank on your car. You have regular old fuel in there and its only goal is to get you from point A to point B, but you also have a reserve can in your trunk, which is filled with premium fuel. However, you can't use it until all of your regular, unleaded fuel is gone. Much like an empty gas tank, there is sludge that can build up on the bottom. This happens when you don't clean your tank out regularly and water and trash start to build up—much like your body when you begin Keto. You are cleaning out the last of the bad 'sludge.' When you are going through the Keto flu, your body is using up the last of its sludge. It's nearly at the point of running out of gas, but not quite yet. It still has enough to run, but barely. Once you run out of the sludge, then you can start using your premium gas. In this case, it is going to be your stored fat. That is the good stuff, and that is when your body jumps out of its depressive, fatigued state. It begins running off of fat instead of carbs and glucose.

Another part of the Keto flu is a mineral deficiency. Because your body is used to having the carbs and glucose run the show, it has a specific process that it goes through to create energy. On the Keto diet, that process has to change. Your body is learning something new and needs time to adapt, much like any other diet. But one thing your body is not doing is regulating sodium and water. It will learn the new steps eventually, but during the Keto flu portion of the diet, it isn't keeping up. Your body is losing a lot of sodium and water all at once. And it's hard to replenish them. Your body is becoming dehydrated. Because your minerals are so low, you are also experiencing an electrolyte deficiency. If you feel nauseous while experiencing the Keto flu, this would be why. The three most important electrolytes to focus on are sodium, of course, magnesium and potassium. There are ways to quickly replenish those electrolytes!

To quickly elevate levels of sodium:
- Bouillon cubes—drop your favorite flavor into a hot cup of water and dissolve it. Each of these could contain upwards of about 2100mg of sodium which is almost half of what you need to make it through the day
- Salt shooter—you could place Himalayan pink salt or a brand of sea salt in a glass of water and mix it with lemon or lime juice.

To quickly elevate levels of Magnesium:
- It is easiest to use a supplement that provides you with your daily need of magnesium.
- Eat avocados!
- Snack on some nuts
- Snack on some seeds

To quickly elevate levels of potassium:
- Eat avocados!
- Eat spinach
- Eat mushrooms

To fully regain all of these electrolytes remember to use an optimal cook method where you are not wasting any of the vital nutrients. If you are cooking mushrooms or spinach, a lot of the nutrients could come out of the broth. So make sure you are eating, and maybe sipping, as much as you can!

Another big part of the Keto flu is caused by the switch from carbs to fats in the gut. When we switch it up, our body begins creating endotoxins because there is too much fat being used at once. Endotoxins are toxins that are present inside of a bacterial cell. It is released when a cell disintegrates which allows them to thrive whereas our gut bacteria has to take a back seat. Endotoxins are also sometimes responsible for mimicking symptoms related to certain diseases. When these endotoxins are released into the bloodstream, the gut bacteria become out of whack and doesn't know what to do in the beginning. The bacteria in our gut is so used to carbs, so once you start throwing fats at it, it has to have time to adapt. The types of bacteria that feed on fat are good, but they have to get ready to thrive.

An easy way to get through this transitional phase of the Keto flu is to drink bone broth. Bone broth is incredibly powerful when it comes to healing the gut. It contains collagen which reduces inflammation and helps heal the intestinal lining. Plus, it's easy for the gut to digest and retain all of its minerals and proteins.

Another part of the Keto flu is your body producing too many Ketones. It is still in its transitional phase and is learning how to adapt to what you are putting into it. The best way to get rid of the excess Ketones is to burn them off. Light cardio is a great way to help your body get through the Keto flu. While transitioning into the Ketogenic state, you and your body have to work together. It makes the Keto flu easier to deal with.

Types of Supplements to Help You on the Ketogenic Diet

There are a number of supplements on the market to help you along on your Keto journey. Supplements are not necessary, but they are helpful when you may not get enough of an electrolyte in your system, or enough of a mineral in your system. They do come in handy. Here are some supplements that might help you.

- Magnesium, potassium, and sodium supplements—these could help you when you are going through the Keto flu. Furthermore, they might become a staple that you take all of the time when you are living your Keto life. It depends on you and how you feel. If your body is low on electrolytes or maybe you know you didn't eat what you needed to eat in a day, these supplements might be a good idea for you.
- Different types of sea salts—if taking a sodium supplement isn't for you, you can experiment with different types of sea salts.
- Fish oil—it puts omega-3 fatty acids into your body that you would normally get from fish. If you are not a fish person, this may work for you. It helps balance those omega-3s and helps to put fat nutrients into the body. Fish oil can aid in weight loss, and for women, it can help with period pains, breast pains, and even pregnancy pains. It's a good general supplement that can make your Keto transition easier.
- MCT oils—these are helpful for the body and to make its job less strenuous. MCT oils are made from coconut oil or palm oil. Coconut is preferred for Keto dieters. But it is an immediate source of Ketones because it glides through the gut into the liver and is either converted into energy or it is converted into Ketones. It also promotes healing to the body.
- Vitamin D—while this one isn't necessary, it is a good idea to have this on hand. Most Americans are Vitamin D deficient. Having a sufficient supply of Vitamin D in your body supports facilitating the absorption of calcium, which is a nutrient that could be lacking in the Ketogenic diet.
- Exogenous Ketones—if there comes a point where you fall off of the Keto diet, this supplement could help you get back into Ketosis faster by providing an outside source of Ketones to your body.

- Keto Green Blend—this could be a number of different things. It is a pill or powder that supplies all (or most) nutritional value that you would otherwise get from leafy green vegetables.

These supplements are just ways to help you succeed on Keto. They aren't necessary, but they are helpful. And some of the help you break out of the Keto flu faster. So, if that is something you are not looking forward to, something like a multivitamin with sodium, magnesium, and potassium could help your transition.

Types of Supplements to Help You Get Over the Ketogenic Flu

These supplements are going to be sort of the same as the Ketogenic Diet Supplements. The same types of supplements that will help you get over Keto flu will aid you on the Ketogenic diet. These include magnesium, potassium, and sodium supplements. MCT oils will help you out as well. You always want to make sure that you are replenishing your body with enough electrolytes and water as your body transitions from carb-burning to fat-burning. You also want to make sure you are drinking a lot of water. The electrolyte supplements are really going to help you overcome the Keto flu. When you begin to feel sick or nauseous it is because you have an electrolyte imbalance. You are quickly losing a lot of your stored nutrients, so you have to make up for it by either taking supplements or eating foods heavy in potassium, magnesium, or sodium. MCT oils are also a great way to begin healing the body. While the body is starting to use Ketones, you can take an MCT oil. It will quickly hit your liver and produce energy or convert to Ketones.

The best 'supplement' you can use is exercise. A light cardio workout is a great tool to help you get over the Keto flu. It doesn't have to be strenuous, but any physical activity will aid you.

Avoid Nutrient-Poor Fat Bombs

Let's refresh on what exactly a fat bomb is and what it is going to do for your body. A fat bomb is essentially a tool to help curb your appetite as you wait for your next meal. They are becoming more popular with the Ketogenic lifestyle as people refrain from eating between meals. These simple, small, circular shaped balls of fat are a great way to avoid over-eating in between meals. Rather than prioritizing protein or other essential nutrients, they prioritize fat, helping you stay full for longer periods of time.

The dangers of fat bombs come into play when you have no self-control. Also, a lot of fat bombs have stuff like nuts in them, which contain a lot of protein. Remember, if you overeat protein it could knock you out of Ketosis. So, putting so much fat and sweetness into a candy-like state could be dangerous. You also want to make sure you are putting the right ingredients into your fat bombs. With these types of 'snacking' foods, you will want to make sure you are really loading up on the fat. These bombs are not supposed to be high in protein. If they are high in protein and fat, it'll take your body even longer to burn the fat that is already inside of your belly or on your butt or thighs. The idea of a fat bomb and why it is so small is because your body can quickly burn off the new fat that just entered, and then continue to burn the rest of the fat that is already there. It is sort of like a jump start. While this is happening, though, you aren't hungry and are hardly thinking about food. This deters you away from snack searching, too. Just grab a fat bomb!

How to Make a Fat Bomb as Nutrient-Dense as Possible?

If you are wanting to make a fat bomb and gain some nutrients while you eat it, there are certain ways to make them. They are a bit more strenuous when it comes to making them, but they are beneficial. These fat bombs can actually be a meal replacement.

First, these fat bombs are more intricate and have more ingredients than the common three or four it takes to make a regular fat bomb.

All fat bombs, though, have a base. Most bases are something that is super high in fat like coconut oil, cream cheese, or butter. On top of the base, you have to add your nutrient-dense ingredients. Herbs and spices are a good way to get some nutrients into your fat bombs. Some spices, like cinnamon, are great antibacterial and immune system healers that could prevent and even treat some infections. Herbs, like rosemary, can boost cognitive function just by the smell. Herbs contain a number of minerals, vitamins, and antioxidants.

Some people even add low carb fruits into their fat bombs. Things such as blueberries, raspberries, and lemon juice are beneficial that protect us from heart diseases, and even cancers.

Nuts and seeds are a great source of protein, fat, and fiber that can be added to your fat bombs. Crushing up nuts or using a nut butter to coat your fat bomb is a great addition because all of the sources of nuts make up a greater body composition and improve health.

Fat bombs don't always have to be sweet in nature. There are great recipes for nutrient-dense fat bombs that taste like pizza, salmon, or jalapeño poppers that act as a meal. These are designed to keep you fuller for a longer period of time.

There is also a thing called bulletproof coffee (BPC). This is a lot like a fat bomb and does the same thing. Grab your favorite coffee. It could be literally any type of coffee you enjoy that does not have carbs or protein. Brew your coffee like you normally would and drop a couple of pads of butter in it. Once it melts, stir it in and drink your coffee as normal. This is a great source of fat in the morning if you are working on your intermittent fasting. It helps fill you up so you curb the need to eat. The same thing can be done with teas, also. It immediately gives you energy! If you do not have butter, MTC oil is a great alternative. It is also preferred by some people because it doesn't have a taste. If neither one of these options are easy for you to get your hands on, coconut oil works and so does heavy cream. Be careful with heavy cream, though. It does contain protein so if you are looking to just stick with fat, heavy cream may not work for you. That protein could be turned into glucose and defeat the purpose of drinking fatty coffee or tea. The body will immediately burn the protein instead of the fat.

The good thing about the Keto diet is that you can find or make any variation of food you normally enjoy, in a low carb fashion. Things like fat bombs are designed to satisfy some of those needs for a pizza, or a cookie.

Chapter 4: How to Find Your Suitable Meal Portion

The easiest way to find a meal portion that is suitable to you and your lifestyle is to first determine your macros. If you find that your macros are too high and that you can't seem to fit it all in a day, then try taking supplements in place of some of the macros you are not reaching. For example, if you are not meeting your protein goal, maybe try a protein powder in a nutrient-dense shake.

There are a number of ways to make sure your meal portions are adequate for the Keto diet. If you find that you can't meet your fat intake, there are simple ways to add the fat into things you normally drink or eat. For example, the BPC is a great way to make sure that the fat gets into your diet. Coffee is something you would normally drink, right? Adding the grass-fed butter or MCT oil will increase your fat intake.

Meal portions are essential in making sure that you enter your correct macros for the day. There are a number of apps that can help with this. MyFitnessPal is a great way to track macros, and it is pretty simple to use. The KetoDiet app is another great way to track your macros. This app also lists recipes by the thousands! So if you are afraid you are not getting enough variety in your diet, this application could be great for you! There are more apps you could download and use. Some of them are listed below.

- Carb Manager
- Total Keto Diet
- Senza
- Cron-O-Meter
- FatSecret
- Wholesome
- Ketosense
- Zero

These apps hold different things as a priority. You should download an app depending on what you think is most important to you. These will help you determine your meal portions. Once you get on a diet, it is hard to figure out what you can and cannot eat. These apps will help you determine your daily intakes. Once you figure that out, you can determine how much you should be eating during what meal. If you have a light breakfast, or no breakfast at all (intermittent fasting), you will be able to eat a heavier dinner or lunch. These meals should meet your daily macros. If you eat a heavy lunch, maybe your dinner is lighter. A majority of your carbs should be eaten in the morning as well, especially before a workout. That way, you are burning them off throughout the day. As a side note, if you eat heavier fats during breakfast or lunch, or maybe a heavy snack, you will find that you are not as hungry at night. Therefore, you'll eat less. Your body will burn stored fat while you sleep rather than the fat you just put into your body.

One of the biggest mistakes made on Keto is thinking that you can just eat lots of meats and cheeses and be okay. That is not the case. A good purchase to keep in mind when starting this diet is measuring cups. To accurately determine macros, you'll need accurate portion sizes. A food scale also works in this circumstance. It will guide you in determining what meal portions are suitable to meet your macros.

Practice Good Eating Habits

It is important to practice good eating habits while on the Ketogenic diet. There are dietitians that stress a couple of key points that will get you further on Keto. But once again, listen to your body. If these habits are not working for you, try something else. The thing about this diet is whatever your body says you need to do, is what you should be doing. This can even mean adding back in a few more carbs per day. Or maybe it is eating more fats. It could even be not eating breakfast in the mornings. Just make sure you are listening to your body's signals. Some of the recommended practices are listed below.

- Eat more fiber — a lot of people do not get enough fiber in their diet.

- Eat greener, above-the-ground vegetables.
- Don't deprive yourself of foods you love. This is very important because a lot of researchers believe if you don't eat what you want when you want it, it will come back to haunt you. So, if you want that chocolate bar, eat it. The good thing about Keto is that you can make a Keto-friendly chocolate bar. You can make almost anything you would normally eat, but it won't mess up your diet.
- Consume a variety of foods — this is also very important. If you find yourself eating the same thing over and over, you will probably become bored. If you become bored, it can really mess with your brain. You want to research a variety of recipes. Almost any food can be made in a Keto-friendly manner. Make sure you shake it up a little, try new foods, and stick to your macros. Plus, if you aren't eating a variety of foods, you may not be getting all of the nutrients you need.
- Control your portions — this can easily happen by eating more fats. You will fill up faster.
- Drink plenty of water — sometimes thirst can be misinterpreted as hunger. Try drinking an 8-ounce glass of water if you start to feel hungry and you know it is not time to eat.
- Pay attention to ingredients and know what you are eating — chances are you've eaten a food in the last couple of days and you have no idea what is in it. If a word ends in -ol, it could be a sugar alcohol. Some Keto dieters do not pay attention to sugar alcohol but some of them have the potential to kick your body out of Ketosis. Not only that, but they can make you crave the real thing!

It is important to know what you are putting into your body. If you aren't familiar with an ingredient, maybe you shouldn't be eating it. Do your research and practice eating habits that work for you and your lifestyle. Also, make sure you are drinking plenty of water. Find different ways to make sure you are eating the right amount of nutrients without overeating or increasing your carbs. It is well worth the time it takes to find what works for you.

Calculate Your Diet Macros

The top macros you will concern yourself with while on the Ketogenic diet are fats, proteins, and carbs. When you first start the Keto diet, it is important to calculate your macros. You have to determine what you are putting into your body, and what your shortcomings are. Once you get used to it, however, it might not be for you. A number of apps will help you figure out what works best for you. They will have you enter your current weight and the weight loss goals you are wanting to achieve. From there, you will be given your daily macro goals. You can enter the foods and drinks you consume in a day and it will let you know what you need to work on. For most people, it is hard to initially consume all of the fats you need to on the Keto diet. Calculating your macros will help! Once you have a good idea of where you stand, or maybe you have reached a weight that you are happy with, you want to maintain it. Then, calculating your macros might not be necessary. Until then, this audiobook will recommend that you do.

Your daily macros may different from someone else on Keto and that is okay. You have to determine what works best for you. Everyone's body composition is different. And depending on the goals you want to achieve, macros will differ for everyone. The general rule is that you need to consume 60% fat, 35% protein, and 5% carbs. This could differ depending on your goals. For example, if you are leaner and you want to retain or grow muscle mass, you would eat less fat than those on a standard Ketogenic diet. Maybe your fat goal for the day is 50%. You would eat a lot more protein, also, because you need to retain your current muscle mass and build on top of it. If you are on the Keto diet to lose more weight, then you would consume more fat than someone who is leaner. It all depends on which Keto diet you are on, and what results you are looking for. Listen the section **"Does the Ketogenic Diet Suit You?"** to fully understand which type of Ketogenic diet you are looking for.

Essential Guide on: Ketogenic Diet for Premenopausal Women

There are a number of problems women face as they become premenopausal. Some of those things are hot flashes, mood swings, insomnia, and weight gain. It is the butt end of comedic relief on some sitcoms but being premenopausal is no laughing matter for women who are going through it. This is the transitional period between when a woman goes from having a regular menstrual cycle to not having one. While this change is happening, hormones are erratic. Once a woman hits menopause, insulin levels and blood glucose imbalances can increase the number of symptoms a woman has. Women are busy trying to find alternative therapies when dealing with these symptoms. Following a standard Ketogenic diet can actually alleviate some of the hard to deal with symptoms.

In a woman's body, hormones act as messengers to the rest of the body to maintain chemical and physical functions of the body. As a women ages, her body produces fewer eggs, progesterone, and estrogen. Changes in these hormones can lead to whacky levels of insulin, ghrelin, and leptin. Having lower levels of estrogen can promote spikes of blood glucose levels as well as insulin resistance. Insulin resistance is a process in which the body's cells resist the effects of insulin. The cells begin to refuse glucose, thus spiking levels of blood sugar. This creates a higher production of insulin. Higher amounts of insulin can potentially result in weight gain.

Because women have been conditioned to refuse fat and stick with a high amount of carbs for numbers of years, it is hard to get on the Keto diet. But the Keto diet can actually help women going through the stages of menopause. It can benefit in many ways. Some of those ways are listed below.

- Can control weight gain
- Reduces the risk of cognitive decline
- Stabilizes blood sugar levels
- Improves mood
- Lowers inflammation
- Increases energy levels
- Improve sleep quality

There are other benefits that come with being on the Keto diet, but these are just a few of the most significant changes that can help a woman's transition to menopause.

Essential Guide on the Ketogenic Diet for Women Who Have Type II Diabetes

Diabetes is a problem with your body as it produces higher levels of glucose than normal. Type II diabetes is the most common form of diabetes. If you have type II, your body does not produce insulin normally. At first, your pancreas produces more to make up for the deficiency, but eventually, the body cannot keep up.

If you have type II diabetes, it is recommended that you begin this diet in the hospital. It is extremely important to monitor your blood glucose and Ketone levels when your body makes the transition and begins burning off the last of its carb fuel. Even once your body adjusts to the diet, it is important to regularly check your glucose levels. Follow up visits to your doctor are also recommended. This is just in case your body is not adapting well to the diet or in case you need to make some adjustments.

There have been a number of studies conducted to see the effects of the Keto diet on people with type II diabetes. Participants of the studies have shown greater control of the glucose in their blood and a need for less medication while on a low carb intake.

Still, this diet may not be what's best for you, if you suffer from type II diabetes. People find that this diet is hard to stay on for long periods of time. Yo-yo dieting (going on and off a diet or switching up diets) can be dangerous for diabetics. If you plan on taking a break from Keto, or maybe trying a different plant-based diet, make sure you talk to your doctor before doing so.

There are a number of benefits that type II diabetics have experienced while using the Keto methods. Participants in other studies saw a reduction in body weight, hemoglobin A1C, and glucose levels in the blood. The low carb diet also shows much more substantial results than a low-calorie diet. While a low-calorie diet has shown improvements, the low carb diet has even greater improvements.

Low-Calorie Diet for People with Type II Diabetes:
- 16% blood glucose reduction
- 2.7% reduction in body mass index
- 6.9 kg reduction of body weight (15.2 pounds)

Low-Carb Diet for People with Type II Diabetes:
- 19.9% blood glucose reduction
- 3.9% reduction in body mass index
- 11.1 kg reduction of body weight (24.4 pounds)

People who had undergone the low carb diet versus the low-calorie diet also found a significant reduction in A1C hemoglobin levels. The reduction of hemoglobin A1C in low carb dieters was over 3 times that of the low-calorie diet (0.5% vs. 1.5%). Hemoglobin A1c is the measure of glucose bound to your red blood cells. If your A1C count is high, you have more glucose in your blood. So, the less, the better. The normal range for a person without diabetes is around 4 and 5.6%. If you have a hemoglobin A1C level between 5.7% and 6.4%, you are at higher risk of becoming diabetic. If your level is above 6.5%, you are considered diabetic. When you test for hemoglobin A1C, and you are diabetic, you want your levels to read less than 7%. The higher your level is, the more you suffer the symptoms typical of being type II diabetic. Type II diabetics that used Keto saw a significant drop in A1C levels. The blood cells live for about three months, so a hemoglobin test every three months showed tests results like this: test one: 7.7%; test 2: 6.4%; test 3: 6.4%; test 4: 6.4%.

Essential Guide on the Ketogenic Diet for Women Who Are Overweight

It is a lot harder for women to lose weight than it is for men, especially when first starting a diet. Women may not see results as fast. This is because of the fact that a woman's body stores more fat than a man's. This is a preemptive design given to women because our bodies are made to birth a child. Fat around the hips and buttocks are produced by estrogen. Stomach fat is usually built because of stress put on the body. Flabby arms could be caused by low testosterone levels. The list goes on, but what does the Ketogenic diet do for these specific types of weight gain?

The process of Ketosis can target specific areas of the body. Ketosis affects a woman's hormones different than a man's. It is a lot harder for a woman to stay in Ketosis because they don't immediately see as much in terms of results. But that doesn't mean it isn't working. Ketosis can help regulate a woman's hormones. There is a lot of hearsay about how a Ketogenic diet can ruin a woman's hormones. This simply isn't true. One of the main concerns is the thyroid. Carbs are necessary for thyroid function. If you lower your carb intake, there is a lot less T3 being circulated throughout the body. The Ketogenic diet does promote a less circulated T3 hormone, but a decreased T3 hormone does not mean your thyroid is dysfunctional or that you are suffering from hyperthyroidism. Hyperthyroidism is categorized by a thyroid not producing enough T4 hormones. It has nothing to do with T3. Thus, the change in the amount of T3 being produced by the thyroid does not cause a dysfunctional thyroid. There is another underlying problem if that is the case. Levels of T3 decrease independently on the Keto diet. A lower level of T3 is actually shown to be beneficial to women. It can preserve muscle longer and improve longevity.

Some women say that Ketosis didn't work for them to lose weight. The answer is simple, though. Those women weren't in Ketosis. So, if you find yourself not losing weight like you want to, or your energy levels are not there, double check your macros. See what you are putting into your body. There is a chance you weren't in Ketosis, to begin with.

Another problem, and one that has already been discussed, is that you might not be eating enough. It is hard for women to eat tons of fat because we have been conditioned to not eat it. So there is a high chance that you simply aren't getting enough into your diet to lose weight.

Another problem that women run into is that they are overtraining. If you work out a lot, a standard Keto diet may not be working for you. Try to find a suitable Keto diet that works with your levels of physical activities. You may need to increase the numbers of carbs you eat per day or increase your protein intake. Overtraining while on Keto can really mess with your hormones. It could also mess with your reproductive organs and increase your levels of cortisol. The problem here is that you are using the wrong tool for the wrong job. So, find something that works for you.

In order to effectively lose unwanted weight, you have to make sure you are in Ketosis, or go-figure, it doesn't work. Women's hormones make it a bit trickier to actually know if the diet is working or not. Find out before giving up and always, always listen to your body.

Chapter 5: How to Get the Best Out of the Ketogenic Diet

Combine the Ketogenic Lifestyle with Exercise to Speed Up Fat Burning.

Trying a new work out when first starting Keto may not be such a good idea. At first, your body is still trying to get used to its new process—hence, you won't feel as great when you are finished. That is not to say that working out is not a part of the Ketogenic diet—it can be. It is important to work out while on Keto (although it is not necessary), but take it easy to start with and don't overwork your body. If you are highly active, don't worry—you can still do Keto.

If you are big into cardio, that is a great way to increase the amount of fat you are burning while on Keto. While you are running or biking, since you are already burning fat, it will oxidize. You will use less oxygen and produce less lactate. This could lead to more fat burning during workouts.

The important thing to remember is that your body needs carbs to boost through a workout, so if you are highly active, try a different Ketogenic diet that allows for a higher carb intake. A common myth that is misunderstood is that you have to work out in order to lose weight on Keto. That is simply not true. The standard Ketogenic diet does not involve working out as a part of the weight loss process—but it can truly help. It can also get you over a plateau. If you hop on a scale every Monday to see how much weight you have lost and see that the number isn't getting any smaller, you may have plateaued. If that is the case, add a simple cardio routine into your day. This could help boost fat burning. Revisiting your macros might help, too.

If you are highly active, don't let the Keto myths scare you away from trying it. It is still a great way to boost energy levels, elevate cognitive brain function, and regulate hormones. Keto also won't make your performance suffer. You might think that because you are eating fewer carbs that you won't have the energy to make it through your run. This is false. It might happen during the start of the Keto diet when your body is making the transition between glucose and fat, but it won't stay that way. Athletes who have been on the Keto diet have had the same performance results as they did before.

The best types of workouts for women on the Keto diet are:

- Cardio (Aerobic exercise): a physical exercise that goes from low to high intensity, lasting over a period of three minutes. An example of this is jogging.

- Anaerobic exercise: a physical exercise that consists of short bursts of energy. For a standard Keto diet, this is not a recommended work out. Fat, alone, cannot fuel this type of activity. An example of this is weight-training.
- Flexibility exercise: This is categorized by the stretching of muscles, joints, and getting a better range of motion in your muscles. An example of this is yoga.

- Stability exercise: This is balance and core training. This helps improve your alignment as well as strengthen muscles. An example of this would be doing squats and liftoffs.

Combine the Ketogenic Lifestyle with Intermittent Fasting.

Intermittent fasting is a big part of Keto. It is an eating style where you only eat in a given time frame and then fast the rest of the time. Most people on Keto fast for 16 hours a day and eat throughout eight hours. For example, you eat only from noon to eight at night. After eight, you do not eat anything and fast while you sleep. Then, you eat again at noon the next day. This is the easiest way to fast. Your body also changes quite a bit during this time. Human Growth Hormones (HGH) increase drastically. When these hormones are deficient in our bodies, it can lead to weight gain and decreased bone mass. So, an increase in HGH is beneficial while on the Keto diet. Insulin sensitivity also improves while fasting. Insulin levels drop dramatically which makes stored body fat easily accessible. Our cells can also go through cellular repair during this time. When cells fast, they start cellular repair processes on other cells that are dysfunctional. They can also digest old proteins that build up inside cells. Fasting can also increase the release of fat burning hormones! Fasting has a host of other benefits. But sometimes fasting isn't for you and that is okay.

If you google fasting for women, you might get a lot of people posting backlash to this method. Everyone is entitled to their own opinions but fasting is not bad like some people think. Women may have to fast differently from men as a result. So, don't accept everything at face value and do your own research to determine whether fasting is right for you. Let's take a look at some of the hormones affected by fasting.

- Starvation hormones: women are much more sensitive to these hormones. It is a protective mechanism in place for bearing a child. If your body realizes it is not receiving adequate foods, it won't want to produce eggs. But this is completely natural. This is why some women drink BPC while fasting. It sends messages to the body to tell it that it is okay and that you are not starving.

- Thyroid hormones: this goes back to the myths about levels of T3 and T4. When you are fasting, the thyroid is less active, but it is also less active during periods of time between meals. It is just the natural response. If you are worried about something being wrong with your thyroid, an easy way to tell is if you become cold all of the time.

If you find that fasting does not work for you, come back to it later and try again. It might not work because your body isn't used to it yet. When you fast, certain processes in the body no longer happen because they don't need to. Sometimes it doesn't work right off the bat. So, revisit it later. It might be easier.

Intermittent fasting revolves around the idea of how our ancestors may not have had food sources readily available to them. The process of hunting and gathering only worked if there were sources of food to hunt and gather. Sometimes, they wouldn't eat for a long period of time. That is when they burnt off their stored fat. Stored fat is a great tool our bodies have used since the beginning. If they didn't have stored fat, we might not be here today! But sometimes, that fat makes us look in a way we don't want to be. We used this ability to survive during periods of famine. Fat was the most sensible way to live during these times. Now that we don't live in periods of famine, the fat just builds until we burn it off.

Chapter 6: Recipes, Advice, and Examples

Quick Breakfast Recipes

If you find yourself busy—maybe you have kids and are trying to get them ready for school in the mornings—these are some easy recipes that will satisfy you (Keto-friendly) and satisfy your family. These are just beginner recipes. Thousands of more recipes can be found online.

Avocado Bacon and Eggs (3g net carbs)

Ingredients:
- **One medium avocado**
- **2 eggs**
- **Bacon bits, or cooked bacon**
- **Salt**
- **Cheddar cheese, shredded**

Instructions:
First, preheat your oven to 425 degrees. Begin by cutting the avocado in half and by removing the pit. You'll want to remove some of the insides of the avocado to make the pit hole bigger. However, don't let the avocado go to waste—eat it! Place your avocado half in a muffin pan to stabilize it while you add the egg to the hole. Sprinkle cheddar cheese on top of the egg, along with salt preference. Cover the top of the avocado with bacon bits. Cook in a muffin pan at 425 degrees for 14–16 minutes. Serve warm. If you do not like bacon, sausage can substitute.

Cheesy Sausage Puffs (1g carb per puff)

Ingredients:
- **1-pound Jimmy Dean Sausage of any variety**
- **2 cups of shredded cheddar cheese**
- **4 eggs**
- **4.5 tbsp. of butter, melted and cooled**
- **2 tbsp. of sour cream**
- **1/3 cup of coconut flour (heaping)**
- **¼ tsp of baking powder**
- **¼ tsp of salt**
- **¼ tsp of garlic (optional)**

Instructions:
Melt butter in the microwave for 10-15 seconds, then place in refrigerator to cool for 10 minutes. Meanwhile, preheat the oven to 375 degrees, and line a large baking sheet with foil, or some sort of non-stick paper. Begin browning the sausage. Once done, drain it and cut it into small pieces. Set aside. In a medium or large size bowl, begin mixing eggs, butter, sour cream, salt, and garlic. Slowly add the coconut flour and baking powder and stir until it is combined. Mix in the browned sausage and cheese. Roll your batter into one-inch balls and place on baking sheet. They only need to be about a half an inch apart from one another. Bake for 14–18 minutes or until lightly browned. Enjoy! Store the leftovers in the freezer for another Keto-friendly breakfast later in the week. Do not keep leftovers longer than 7 days. If you are craving a bread-like consistency, add another half a cup of coconut flour to make them a bit more bread-like.

Keto Blackberry Cheesecake Smoothie (6.7g net carbs)

Ingredients:
- ½ a cup of blackberries, fresh or frozen
- ¼ cup of full-fat cream cheese, or creamed coconut milk
- ¼ cup of heavy whipping cream or coconut milk
- ½ cup of water
- 1 tbsp. of MCT oil or extra virgin coconut oil
- ½ tsp of sugar-free vanilla extract or ¼ tsp of pure vanilla powder
- Optional: 1-3 drops of liquid stevia or another artificial, Keto-approved sweetener

Instructions:

Combine all ingredients into a blender with the exception of the blackberries. Add the stevia if you would like to. Slowly blend all ingredients together. Once blended, add in blackberries slowly. Continue adding blackberries until ½ a cup is reached. Blend to preferred consistency. Pour in a glass and enjoy!

Quick Recipes for Lunch

Cheesy Cauliflower and Bacon Soup (4.4g net carbs)

Ingredients:
- 1/4 cup of olive oil
- 1 tsp minced garlic
- 1 medium head of cauliflower, chopped
- 2 cups of chicken broth
- 1 cup of water
- 1 cup of heavy whipping cream
- 1 tsp xanthan gum
- 1.5 cups of shredded cheddar cheese
- 4 tbsp. bacon bits

Instructions:
In a deep stove-top pan, heat up ¾ of the olive oil and minced garlic. Once it is hot, add in the medium head of cauliflower, chopped. Keep on high heat. Pour in chicken broth and water and wait for a boil. Stir frequently. Once it is boiling, add in the heavy whipping cream and continue to stir. Bring the heat down to medium. In another bowl, mix the excess olive oil and xanthan gum together until blended. Drop your mixture into the rest of the soup and continue to stir. It should start thickening. Slowly add in your cheese so it has a chance to melt. Pour your bacon bits in, serve, and enjoy!

Chili Lime Lettuce Wraps *(1.9g net carbs per leaf)*

Ingredients:

Marinade:
- 2 tbsp. of olive oil
- 1 tbsp. of white wine vinegar
- Zest from 2 limes
- 2 tbsp. lime juice
- 1 clove of garlic, pressed
- ½ tsp of chili powder
- ¼ tsp of salt
- ½ tsp of paprika
- ¼ tsp of stevia
- 1 tbsp. of cilantro

For Chicken:
- 1 ½ tbsp. of butter
- ½ pound of chicken breast, cut into bite-sized pieces

For Aioli:
- 3 tbsp. of mayo
- Zest from lime
- 1 tsp of lime juice
- ½ a tsp of finely chopped cilantro
- 1 garlic clove, pressed

For Lettuce Wraps:
- 3 large lettuce leaves

Instructions:
In a medium-sized bowl, add all of the marinade ingredients together and blend them together until you feel they are evenly incorporated. Put the small cuts of chicken into a dish for marinating. Pour the marinated mixture over the chicken and make sure all sides of the chicken pieces have been coated evenly. Cover the dish and put in the fridge for 1–2 hours to marinate. In a saucepan, melt the butter on low heat. Once the

butter is completely melted, add in the marinated chicken and turn to medium-high heat. Allow the chicken to brown on one side before flipping it to another side. The chicken can be cooked in different batches, also. For the aioli, combine all ingredients into a small bowl until evenly mixed together. Next, take your lettuce leaves and dispense chicken evenly on each leaf with a spoon. On top of the chicken, place the desired amount of aioli sauce. Serve, and enjoy!

Keto Philly Cheesesteak Omelet (4.9g carbs per two omelets)

Ingredients:
- **4 large eggs**
- **2 tbsp. of olive oil**
- **1 ounce of yellow onion, sliced**
- **½ medium green bell pepper, sliced**
- **¼ pound shaved ribeye**
- **1 tsp salt**
- **½ tsp of pepper**
- **2 ounces of provolone cheese, sliced thin**

Instructions:
Gently whisk eggs and ½ of the olive oil in a medium bowl. Heat a medium non-stick skillet and pour half of the egg mixture into it. Cover until the egg is cooked all of the ways through. Use a spatula to release the edges of the omelet from the skillet and put on a plate. Repeat the same process with the rest of the egg mix. Once the other egg is done, pour rest of the olive oil into the same skillet. Pour in sliced green peppers and onions into the pan. Cook on a medium heat until onions begin to caramelize, and the green peppers turn soft. Remove these items from the pan and set them aside. Season the ribeye with salt and pepper. Sauté meat over medium heat or until cooked all the way through. Add pepper and onion mixture back into the pan with the meat to heat back up if necessary. Take your omelet shells and layer provolone cheese and the hot mixture of meat and veggies on top. Serve, and enjoy!

Zucchini Crust Grilled Cheese

Ingredients:
- **4 cups of zucchini, shredded**
- **1 large egg**
- **½ cup of shredded mozzarella cheese**
- **4 tbsp. of grated parmesan cheese**
- **1 tsp dried oregano**
- **½ tsp of salt**
- **Black pepper**
- **1 tbsp. of butter**
- **1/3 cup of shredded cheddar cheese, room temperature**

Instructions:
Heat your oven to 450 degrees. Place a rack in the middle of the oven. Line a large baking sheet with parchment paper and grease it with butter, liberally. Place zucchini in microwave on high for six minutes. Once it is done, transfer it to a tea towel and squeeze out as much liquid as you can. This is super important because if you don't drain the zucchini, you'll end up with a mushy grilled cheese. It becomes almost impossible to use as slices of bread. In a large bowl, mix zucchini, egg, mozzarella cheese, parmesan cheese, oregano, salt, and pepper (to taste). Spread the zucchini mixture onto the lined baking sheet and shape it into four squares. Bake the zucchini for 15–20 minutes or until the squares become lightly brown. Remove from the oven and let it cool for about 10 minutes. Be careful during this step, you don't want to break the bread. Heat a skillet over medium heat. Butter one side of each of the zucchini bread. Place one slice of bread in the pan, buttered side down. Sprinkle with cheese. Place another slice of zucchini bread on top, buttered side up. Cook until golden brown on the first side. Flip and do the same with the other side. Each side should brown in 2–4 minutes. Cut, serve and enjoy!

Quick Dinner Recipes

Broiled Salmon (<1g carb per 1 oz. of salmon)

Ingredients:
- **4 (4 oz.) salmon filets**
- **1 tbsp. of grainy mustard**
- **2 cloves garlic, finely minced**
- **1 tbsp. finely minced shallots**
- **2 tsp finely chopped thyme leaves**
- **2 tsp fresh rosemary**
- **Juice of half of a lemon**
- **Salt, to taste**
- **Pepper, to taste**
- **Lemon slices, for serving**

Instructions:
Heat broiler and line a large baking pan with parchment paper. Place salmon on the pan. In a small bowl mix together the ingredients (mustard, garlic, shallots, thyme, rosemary, lemon juice, salt, and pepper). Spread mixture all over salmon fillets. Broil 7–8 minutes. Garnish with lemon slices and fresh thyme (if you'd like) and serve. Enjoy!

Taco Cheese Cups (1g carb per cup)

Ingredients:
- 3 ½ cups of shredded cheddar cheese
- 1 tbsp. of extra virgin olive oil
- 1 onion, chopped
- 3 cloves of garlic, minced
- 1 pound of ground beef
- 1 tsp chili powder
- ½ tsp ground cumin
- ½ tsp paprika
- Salt
- Chopped tomatoes, for serving
- Diced avocado, for serving
- Sour cream, for serving
- Chopped cilantro, for serving

Instructions:
First, preheat the oven the 375 degrees. Line a large baking pan with parchment paper. Put tablespoons of cheddar cheese in a small pile on the baking sheet. Bake until the cheese becomes bubbly and the edges become golden. Let them cool for a minute after removing from the over. Grease the bottom of a muffin pan and carefully peel the cheese off of the parchment paper. Place them inside the muffin tins. Let them cool for about ten minutes. In a large skillet, heat on medium, heat up the extra virgin olive oil. Add the onions and let them sauté for about five minutes, or until they become soft and slightly transparent. Add the garlic and ground beef next. Cook the beef until it is no longer pink. This will take about 6 or 7 minutes. Once that is done, drain the beef and place it back in the skillet. Add the paprika, cumin, chili powder, and salt. Transfer the cheese cups to a serving plate. Fill them with the ground beef, then add the tomatoes, sour cream, avocado, and cilantro. Serve, and enjoy!

Chicken Zucchini Alfredo (4g net carbs per serving)

Ingredients:
- 3 large zucchinis
- 2 tbsp. extra virgin olive oil
- ¾ pounds of chicken breast
- Salt
- Pepper
- 1 tsp Italian seasoning
- 2 cloves of garlic, finely minced
- ¾ cup half and half
- 4oz cream cheese
- ½ cup of freshly grated parmesan
- ¼ cup of chopped parsley

Instructions:
Make zucchini "pappardelle." Using a vegetable peeler, peel the zucchinis to make long, thin strips. Lay them on a paper-towel-lined baking sheet until ready to use them. On medium heat, place the chicken breast and one tablespoon of extra virgin olive oil in a large skillet and let it cook 6–8 minutes on each side. Season each side of the chicken with salt, pepper, and Italian seasoning. Transfer the chicken to a cutting board. Slice it into strips. Add the remaining tablespoon of extra virgin olive oil to the skillet. Add the garlic and cook it until it becomes fragrant. This usually takes about a minute. From there, add the half and a half and the cream cheese to the skillet. Stir this often until the cream cheese becomes melted. Add in the freshly grated parmesan, season with salt and pepper. Wait for the sauce to thicken (about 3 to 5 minutes). Finally, fold in the chicken and zucchini pappardelle. Add the parsley last. Serve and enjoy immediately!

Easy Turkey Chili (5.5g carbs)

Ingredients:
- 1 tbsp. of virgin olive oil
- 1 yellow onion, diced
- 1 small green pepper, diced
- 2 cloves of minced garlic
- 2 pounds of ground turkey breast
- 1.5 tbsp. of chili powder
- 1 tsp of garlic powder
- 1 tbsp. ground cumin
- 1 tsp cayenne powder
- 1 cup low carb tomato sauce
- Salt and pepper, to taste
- Shredded cheddar cheese, for serving
- Sour cream, for serving

Instructions:
Heat a large skillet with the olive oil in it. Heat should be on medium high. Add in the diced onions and peppers and sauté until they are browned. This should take about 3–4 minutes. Stir in the garlic and cook for about another minute or so. Add in the ground turkey and season it with salt and pepper. Cook the turkey until it is completely browned and then add in the other seasonings. Stir in the tomato sauce and season to taste if what you have already added is not enough. Simmer on low heat for ten minutes. Serve with shredded cheese and sour cream. Enjoy!

Advice

Beginning the Keto diet can be really hard, especially if it is already hard for you to find time to eat a good, nutritional meal. But before you inlay the idea, look up some success stories. See how other women in your position have successfully done Keto and managed to keep everything else intact. It makes your journey a lot easier. You can also ask for help. Having someone support your journey—maybe a spouse or your children—can push you to do your absolute best. It helps keep you motivated!

A lot of women revolve their Keto diets around foods that they know they love. I think the love of pizza, cheeseburgers, and pasta are a common factor between us all. The good thing about these and many other foods is that there is a Keto-version of them. You can have foods you really want and still eat healthily. If we could all make the switch, I think we would be surprised at how good the food really is.

Another great way to be at your *Keto-best* is to connect with people on social media. Putting yourself out there is a little intimidating, but you would be surprised at how many people are going through the same thing you are going through. You both could help each other out. Talking about what problems you are having warrants an array of answers from people all over the world. Within those people, there could be someone who is just like you–boost each other up and get healthy!

Women Who Gladly Shared Their Keto Stories Online

Allison, 41, lost 25lbs in 6 months: Find some high-protein recipes you love!
"My current favorite is stuffed peppers with ground beef and melted mozzarella. And low carb desserts are key! They kept me from feeling deprived. I used resources like Keto cookbooks."

Esther, lost 41lbs in 5 months: Eat at least 50 grams of protein a day!

"In the past, diets have left me crazy-hungry. Now, I maintain a caloric deficit, but I do it while making sure I have enough fat, protein, and fiber, which keeps me satisfied."

Joanna, 33, lost 60lbs in a year: Eat the Keto-friendly foods that you legit enjoy!
"I built my diet around foods that I really like: Caesar salads, cheese, and chicken wings. I stopped feeling guilty about eating them (which I did in the past because they're high in fat) and now I actually take pleasure in the food that I'm eating. The best part is that my cravings have pretty much stopped."

Success stories are everywhere! You have the potential to be one of them—if you want to. The most important thing to remember is that your body is the most important thing. If your body isn't happy, you aren't either. Listen to what your body is telling you. Also, don't fear away because of myths! Our bodies used to run perfectly fine, as they would on the Keto diet—way, way, way back in the day. The Keto diet is designed around how the first people lived without a grocery store or farming. All they had to eat was what they could find. Hence, if they didn't hunt and gather, they didn't eat. If they got a rabbit, they would fuel their bodies with what fat, protein, and fiber they could gain that. Sometimes, they would have to go days without eating, and that is why intermittent fasting is an intricate detail of the Keto diet. You will function normally on this diet, but be aware of the Keto flu. It is short-lived, but it can take its toll on your body. There are steps to help you get past it easier.

- Some advice to get through the Keto flu is to eat an excessive amount of fat for the first week or so. Let your body know things are changing!
- Don't restrict calories! Eat until you are not hungry anymore.
- Keto or Fasting-Choose one to start! You don't have to do both, and you definitely don't have to stick with whichever is not working for you.
- If you make fat bombs, make them as nutrient-dense as possible.

- Don't be hard on yourself if you don't meet your daily goals.
- Be aware of the low-protein slippery slope—high levels of Ketones don't mean much if you are losing muscle instead of fat.
- Create a rewards system—if you make your macros for a couple of days, maybe have an extra fat bomb the next morning!
- Don't treat yourself with a cheat day! This is a big one. Having one cheat day will not be worth the body being knocked out of Ketosis. It will be like going through the Keto flu all over again once you get back on track. Reward with fats, not carbs!
- Set realistic goals, not ones that will make you feel like you need to be punished for not reaching them.
- Track everything you put into your body!
- Add in exercise if you feel like doing so!

There are a number of different ways to keep yourself on track. Do your best if the Keto diet is for you. If it isn't right now, that is okay. Maybe come back to it at another time. If you are wanting a weight change or wanting an immediate change to how you feel, the Keto diet could be a perfect fit. If you find yourself getting bored, switch up your meal plans! Maybe creating new goals for yourself. Experience the lifestyle change that is the Ketogenic diet. You'll be glad you did!

Here is a beginner's food list. These are the essential products you'll need to begin Keto. They are high in fat, protein, and low in carbs. Some of them are used purely for the cooking method.

- Salmon
- Sardines
- Cod liver oil
- Eggs
- Grass-fed beef
- Grass-fed butter
- Grass-fed ghee

- Hemp seeds
- Chia Seeds
- Flax seeds
- Stevia
- Allulose
- Monk fruit
- Erythritol
- Spinach
- Zucchini
- Broccoli
- Cauliflower
- Lettuce
- Mushrooms
- Kale
- Garlic
- Celery
- Blackberries
- Raspberries
- Strawberries
- Avocados
- Eggplant
- Squash
- Lemon
- Lime
- Tomatoes
- Olives
- Peppers
- Cucumbers
- Coconut
- Cheese
- Heavy whipping cream
- Cream cheese
- Sour cream
- Plain Greek yogurt
- Nut milk
- Cottage cheese

- Olive oil
- Avocado oil
- MCT oil
- MCT powder
- Coconut oil
- Walnut oil
- Ricotta
- Wild-caught seafood
- Wild-caught game
- Uncured bacon
- Bone Broth
- Apple cider vinegar
- Dark chocolate (high percentage of cocoa)

This is, by all means, not a complete list of grocery items for Keto. But most of these items will get you started. Make sure you read labels before you purchase these items. Some products have additives to make the products last longer. You want the most whole foods you can get. Also, watch out for sugar alcohols!

This may look like an expensive list—and depending on where you live, it might be. However, the good news about this list is that it can last you for a long time. For example, buying a box of stevia or buying any of the cooking oils is going to last you for more than one meal. It can actually last weeks! Other things—you can divide up. Ground-fed beef can be stretched out for a couple of meals. If you and your family are fans of leftovers, you can really stretch it out. Things like heavy whipping cream—you might have to purchase more often, as it gets consumed pretty quickly. Other things like the leafy greens and berries are more of the same. But luckily, you are on Keto, and you will be consuming them rather quickly to meet your macros! A typical day of eating a standard Keto diet can look like this:

Breakfast:
- 3 large eggs cooked with grass-fed butter
- 1 medium avocado topped with sea salt
- 4oz of smoked salmon
- Ghee – 2 tbsp.

Lunch:
- 1 can of tuna
- Raw spinach with two tablespoons of olive oil
- Raw almonds

Dinner:
- 1 tablespoon of butter
- 2 cups of mushrooms
- Grilled chicken leg with skin

These items will use a lot of the products you bought on your list. You will also have a lot of leftovers to use for your next meal. Hence, while the first shopping trip might be a bit expensive, it won't stay that way. The next few trips to the store will be to replenish your vegetables and dairy-based products. This typical day will also differ a bit depending on your macros. Therefore, this may work for some people—but if your goals on Keto are different, you may need to increase fat intake a bit more or maybe consume a bit more protein. It also depends on which Keto diet you are doing. If you are, for example, doing the high-protein Ketogenic diet, then your protein intake will be a lot higher than a person who is doing a standard Ketogenic diet (SKD). If you are on a CKD, then your carb intake will be higher. The same goes for a TKD, which allows for more carbs based on your workouts.

Conclusion

Thank you for making it through to the end of Keto Diet for Women: Beginner's Guide to Loss Weight Fast. Let's hope it was informative and able to provide you with all of the tools you need to achieve your goals—whatever they may be.

The next step is to determine if the Ketogenic Lifestyle is for you. If it is, please refer to this audiobook as your one-stop information shop. Everything that you need to know is here! If you are a woman who is premenopausal, suffering from type II diabetes, or just want to lose weight—your answers are here. There are essential details on how to go through the Keto diet as a woman. You'll find great, easy recipes to start your new life with as well as some key snacks that will help you make it through the day. It's all here!

Thank you.

INTERMITTENT FASTING FOR WOMEN

Have You Heard of The Multiple Benefits of Intermittent Fasting but Don't Know Where to Start? Learn Fasting's Best Kept Secrets & Maximize Weight Loss in Just 30 Days

Table of Contents

Introduction

Welcome to the world of intermittent fasting!

Intermittent fasting simply means not eating for a designated period of time or a set number of hours and then eating during a time restricted feeding period. While the act of fasting has been around thousands of years, in the last several years, more and more women are engaging in the lifestyle of intermittent fasting. Intermittent fasting is proving to be highly beneficial to women health. There are countless benefits to participating in the lifestyle. Unlike the traditional diet, it focuses more on when you eat as opposed to what you eat. There are many ways to use fasting to your benefit and various techniques.

In recent culture, intermittent fasting has become increasingly popular. There has been research to support the practice. There is evidence of benefits on many body systems including slowing down aging, better cardiac health, better focus, weight loss, and multiple other benefits. While the vast majority of women are interested in intermittent fasting for the aid in weight loss, this guide goes over the other perks of the lifestyle, as well. Unfortunately, there is some negative stigma surrounding intermittent fasting. We have been programmed to think we need to eat six meals a day and be constantly snacking. Sadly, this is based on old, outdated science. More recent science has shown quite the opposite. There are numerous recent studies that show how effective intermittent fasting can be for your overall health. There are many different types of fasting with each having their own benefits.

This guide is to help you decide which fasting protocol is best for you and to help you understand how it works, the common myths, struggles and benefits, as well as guidelines for practices that can aid you in fasting and help you to be successful if and when you choose to endeavor into the program of intermittent fasting. There is information about special circumstances and intermittent fasting such as pregnancy, PCOS, diabetes, and for weight loss as well as tools and tricks to help you get through your hunger and onto the roads of a healthier lifestyle!

Chapter One

The History of Intermittent Fasting

Fasting has been around nearly as long as mankind itself. There are many old written sources that have shown that "starvation" has been used in various cultures, countries, and ancient civilizations to help the body recover and restore itself. It seems they were taking advantage of the benefits long before modern times. Ancient India, Greece, and Rome, in particular, used intermittent fasting, not only to strengthen the body but also to help prevent diseases. Back in ancient times, when hunting and berry gathering was one of the main sources of food, there were periods of time where nothing could be found, so natural fasting took place. Involuntary fasting caused the hunters and gatherers to be inadvertently and greatly strengthened by the gaps in sustenance. The ancient Greeks particularly believed medical treatments and cures could be found and were observed in nature. When humans, dogs, cats, and most animals are sick, they do not want to eat. This is considered the internal physician in some cultures; it is believed that the body is instinctually fasting to help to heal its self. The ancient Greeks also believed fasting helped to improve mental and cognitive function. This makes sense if you think about when you eat a big meal and feel sleepy and tired or have "food coma" as many like to call it, versus when you are fasting and your brain hyper-focuses on the task at hand. The practices of controlled starvation are key in many of the world's religions, proving self-control, and penitence. Many religions practice fasting for periods such as Ramadan in the Islamic culture where they do not eat from sunup to sundown. Christianity recognizes the forty days of lent, which represents the time that Jesus Christ fasted. Fasting is recognized in Islamic religions, Buddhism, Christianity, and countless others.

Ramadan is an Islamic tradition that is practiced by Muslims. During Ramadan, they fast during the daylight hours, finally eating only once the sun has set. While it sounds terrible at first, many reports they actually feel better after a few days of the practice. This is because they adjust to the schedule and their bodies learn to adapt to no food for a time period. This is exactly what intermittent fasting is about.

However, in more recent years, there has been scientific research discovering and confirming the various benefits of intermittent fasting for women. Science is now beginning to prove what was already known in ancient times. The multiple and seemingly endless benefits keep climbing. The benefits include slowing down the aging process, sharper focus, weight loss, better cardiac health, there is evidence it both reduces the chances of cancer and helps your body to fight it off and a wide range of other advantages, with little consequences to the practice.

Studies on Mice and Rats

There have been a growing number of studies done on mice and rats that show rather promising results with intermittent fasting. They have shown evidence of decreased aging with better stem cell rejuvenation. The studies have shown good results with fighting certain cancers by helping to better target the immune response and there have been various other studies involving weight loss and diabetic patients. Generally, mice and rats have very similar anatomy and organ systems as humans. Since our systems are so similar to mice and rats, the good results in the lab animals is a very good sign that there will be positive results in humans as well.

How Intermittent Fasting Works and Why It Is Healthy

All intermittent fasting means, in the simplest terms, is that you go through an extended period without eating. It can range from a few hours to several days. Most people stick to fasts that last somewhere between twelve and twenty hours. The time you are not eating or fasting is known as your fasting window. The time that you are not fasting is called your feeding period.

The fasting window is only for drinking water, black coffee, herbal teas, and sparkling water; any beverages with sugar, fat, or additives will break the fast. Especially starting out, it is important to maintain a fast for the time period that was set. When you consume food or eat a meal, your body spends several hours processing the meal you just ate, burning what it can from the food you consumed. Because you just ate food, it is easy to burn, and an available energy for it to break down. Your body will break down the food you just consumed instead of the fat you already have stored. This is especially true if you have just eaten food with a lot of sugar and carbohydrates. Sugars and carbs are easy to break down and convert into energy.

While you are on a fast, your body is more likely to break down and convert to energy the fat your body already has stored, as you are no longer giving it simple easy fuel. When you are in a fast, your body naturally lowers its blood sugar and insulin levels. The lower your insulin is, the less you will feel hungry and the less you will crave food. There are other reasons why intermittent fasting is considered healthy. It naturally strengthens the body and helps it to fight diseases more efficiently. Intermittent fasting also has many effects on the body systems, glands, and hormones. Most of them being positive effects. There has been evidence of fasting helping diabetics naturally regulate their insulin as well as many positive metabolic effects. To put it in the simplest terms, intermittent fasting works so well because it encourages the body into a state of ketosis, where it is burning the fat that it already has stored instead of newly consumed foods for energy. This is also what makes intermittent fasting healthy and beneficial. The best part is it is a lifestyle more than it is a diet, as it does not restrict what you eat, just the time period that you are eating.

The Hormones, Systems, and Organs Involved and Affected in Intermittent Fasting

To understand how intermittent fasting works, it is important to understand the major hormones and body systems that are affected by it. Several of the metabolic hormones are involved in a period of fasting as well as when you end a fast. These hormones include insulin, leptin, ghrelin, the human growth hormone, and several other hormones, organs, glands, and systems. Each hormone has a different purpose and they all come together to create the metabolism. Most women prefer a fast metabolism as that promotes a lower weight. Intermittent fasting is known for helping the metabolism and hormones self-regulate for a healthier body overall.

- The metabolism and intermittent fasting.

The metabolism is essentially a word used to describe the series of chemical reactions involved in sustaining life, in any and all organisms. There are three major purposes of the metabolism. These purposes are converting food into fuel so that cellular processes can adequately run, converting fuel and food into building blocks for proteins, lipids, and nucleic acids, and the elimination of nitrogenous wastes. The metabolism is basically the sum of all the chemical reaction that occurs in the body and include digestion and transporting substances from one cell to another.

A common misconception with intermittent fasting is that it significantly slows down the metabolism. Shockingly enough, however, there is some more recent research that suggests that intermittent fasting has the same or less negative effects on the metabolism when compared to regular, traditional dieting. The reasoning behind the belief that intermittent fasting helps to improve the metabolism is that there is less lean body mass loss, and the body enters the phase of fat burning. While it is not possible to lose weight without losing some amount of lean body mass, fewer seemed to be lost with intermittent fasting as opposed to traditional calorie and carb restricting diets. To preserve more of the body's lean body mass, the calorie burning of the body slows down some. Short fasting periods, however, encourage the body to tap into its own fat stores and burn a larger amount of fat stores and mass for energy. Basically, it seems that there are two major factors that make intermittent fasting compatible with most metabolisms. One being that the fasting is indeed intermittent, meaning no more than a day and that you are still providing the body with adequate nutrition in the feeding windows.

- Insulin — the 'feed me' hormone.

Our body systems react to consuming food (energy consumption) by producing insulin. Insulin is a hormone produced by the pancreas that regulates the amount of glucose in the blood. The more you eat, especially carbs and sugar, the more insulin your body produces and the less your body converts its own fats to energy. It is important for your body to be sensitive to insulin as the more sensitive your body is to the hormone, the more efficiently you will be able to use the food you consume. Insulin is also the hormone that tells you are hungry. So frequently people are feeding the cycle of eating, and then the insulin tells your body that it is hungry when really it does not need food at that time. Staying sensitive to insulin is vital maintaining a good rhythm in your fasting protocol. Once you have adjusted to intermittent fasting, your body's insulin will naturally be lowered and will stabilize. Once your insulin stabilizes, you will feel hungry much less often. Many women have stated that the first several days were difficult but after that, they simply stopped feeling hungry. All these effects are because of the natural regulation of the body's insulin. Keeping insulin lowered naturally is also proving to be extremely beneficial to type two diabetic patients. They are able to control their insulin much better simply by adjusting when they eat.

- Leptin — the 'stop eating' hormone.

Leptin is another hormone affected in intermittent fasting. Leptin is the hormone that tells you when to stop eating. Low leptin leads to an increase in hunger, which can lead to easily overeating. Generally, slender or lean individuals have low levels of leptin while heavy or obese individuals have high levels of leptin. The trouble with having high levels of leptin chronically is that leptin resistance develops. Much like insulin resistance develops when someone has chronically high insulin. When evaluated long-term, leptin is regulated by the total amount of fat mass in the body. A sharp drop in leptin can also have a poor effect on other hormones, and the rate of your metabolism in general. Intermittent fasting helps to regulate and encourage healthy levels of leptin, so it will become easier to maintain a healthy metabolism.

- Blood Glucose

Blood glucose is also known as blood sugar and is a hormone that is a simple sugar. Blood glucose is stored in the liver and skeletal system and is considered a primary energy source in the human species. Blood glucose is vital to the proper function of various organs, most importantly the brain. The brain alone can consume up to sixty percent of glucose in a fasted individual. The human body cannot use blood glucose as energy, so when enough insulin is not produced, the body converts its already stored fat into energy. A ketogenic diet is based on hypoglycemia or when your body is running on low blood sugar. This keeps the body constantly burning fat which results in the often-desired weight loss and lower fat mass in the body.

- Ghrelin — the 'you fed me at this time yesterday' hormone.

Ghrelin is a tricky little hormone that is responsible for telling your body to eat at the same time every day. With intermittent fasting, your ghrelin levels have to adjust and stabilize, which can often take a few days. Ghrelin is also sometimes responsible for making people irritable or 'hangry' while they are adjusting to the altered hormone levels. The best thing to remind yourself when struggling to regulate is that it will pass.

- The Human Growth Hormone

The human growth hormone (HGH) is increased when intermittent fasting protocols are engaged in the body. It has been proven that they can increase as much as five times the average. When the human growth hormone is increased, it produces more blood glucose, which helps to control hunger more easily. The human growth hormone helps with many body functions and the excess that intermittent fasting causes are beneficial in many ways. The human growth hormone can also actually speed up body repair as well. Because the human growth hormones drive muscle synthesis, it helps to speed up the healing process and allows you to recover from workouts and injuries quicker.

- Female hormonal effects.

There is some controversy surrounding the effects of intermittent fasting on the female hormones. One potential consequence is that intermittent fasting can "turn off" the ovaries and the reproductive hormones. When you look at the human female body objectively, it is designed for reproduction. When you practice intermittent fasting and reach a fat burning state, it sometimes causes the reproductive system to shut off temporarily. The body realizes that it is using up the fat reserves and tells the reproductive system that it is not being fed correctly and that it is therefore not suitable for childbirth. This can stop a woman's menstrual cycle. Even though you know in your mind that you will eat again, on a cellular and hormonal level, your body does not know that, so it engages in this survival mode. This does not happen to all women and if you begin missing your periods, you should consider adjusting your fasting and feeding cycles. It is always wise to discuss with a physician as well. Early onset menopause caused by this phenomenon is not something that should be taken lightly. Early onset menopause is one of the few occurrences that can happen that may mean the intermittent fasting lifestyle is not compatible with your body and reproductive system.

- The thyroid and intermittent fasting.
Intermittent fasting can have both positive and negative effects on the thyroid. The thyroid is a gland, located in the neck, that is responsible for secreting hormones that regulate the growth rate and metabolism in humans.

Women with hypothyroidism or low thyroid originally were warned to stay away from intermittent fasting and food depravation lifestyles. Recent research has shown this to be false, however. In the recent studies, it has shown that even on long-term fast, like for seven to ten days, there are not any real negative effects. However, many doctors and scientist do believe that what really affects hypo thyroids is the calorie intake. With too low of calories, the thyroid begins to struggle which means that intermittent fasting is okay for hypothyroidism because it is not actually restricting the calorie intake, just changing the intake times. While fasting can be a stress on our body, especially before it has fully adjusted to intermittent fasting, there is no recent research supporting that it is bad for those women with thyroid issues. The thyroid is a fairly sensitive gland and can cause many symptoms when it is not functioning properly. Often, the root causes of thyroid issues could be autoimmune, lack of proper nutrients that help the thyroid, increased stress hormones and cortisol can also exasperate the thyroid functions, the infection can affect the thyroids as well as poor digestion. Low stomach acid and low enzymes can affect it as well. Essentially, if you have a thyroid issue and want to engage in intermittent fasting, it is generally okay if you follow the simple guidelines. These include getting enough nutrition and calories and making sure your digestive system is adequate.

For a healthy thyroid, fasting does not negatively affect the thyroid. Thyroid hormones, one of them being T3. T3 is the active form of thyroid. It is actually one of the hormones responsible for regulating certain functions of your body. T3 is responsible for your heart rate, some components of your metabolism, and your body temperature. T4 is a prohormone. T4 is the main hormone secreted by the thyroid. T4 is important because it actually encourages the production of the T3 hormone. Then there is also TSH, or the thyroid stimulating hormone, that encourages the production of both T3 and T4. When the thyroid stimulating hormone is high, it means the body is having a hard time producing T3. After a study that was a ten-day fast, there was evidence of a slight change in the T3 hormone, however, there was none what so ever in the T4 hormone and no change in the TSH or thyroid stimulating hormone. What this meant, in the end, is that a long ten day fast messed with the active thyroid hormone a little bit, but the long-term effect was unchanged. So, all it really did was temporarily slow down the metabolism in the state of a fast. The multi-day fast changed the active thyroid but did not ultimately damage or change the ability to make T4 or TSH. What this means is that all it did was slow down the metabolism but only while they were actually fasting. Not during the time of feeding. Once the fast is broken, it actually wakes up the metabolism so fast that it compensates for slowing down during the period of fasting. Therefore, in the end, the study showed the compensation increased the metabolism. The bottom line is, while the thyroid hormones are affected during intermittent fasting, it is not necessarily negative or harmful and can actually help to speed up the metabolism.

The Hidden Benefits of Intermittent Fasting

While most people like the idea of intermittent fasting for weight loss purposes, there are numerous benefits that are not as well-known and talked about as well. To name just a few, there is the natural regulation of insulin and blood sugar (glucose); intermittent fasting helps to reduce risks of common diseases like heart disease, obesity, and diabetes; intermittent fasting helps to actually slow the body's aging; and it has been known to drastically improve focus and energy. This is especially true while on a fast. Many women have stated that their focus has never been better than it has been while mid fast.

- Benefit One: Intermittent fasting helps to naturally regulate the body's insulin and blood sugar levels.

This concept has recently had a fair amount of attention because of the great results in diabetic patients. They are able to naturally regulate their insulin levels while using intermittent fasting. This has shown to work as well, if not better than just controlling the diet and exercise. Many type two diabetics were able to use intermittent fasting solely as their means of controlling the condition.

- Benefit Two: Helps to reduce risks of very common diseases such as obesity, heart disease, and diabetes and helping to strengthen the body.

Intermittent fasting forces the body into ketosis which is also a state of fat burning. Since the body is burning fat, it is decreasing the risk factors for common diseases. Being in a fat burning state helps to release certain chemicals into the bloodstream that help to break up the bad cholesterol. The insulin is naturally lowered and regulated for diabetics and weight loss is promoted and generally achieved by the forced state of fat burning. Helping reduce illness and diseases is an age-old claim to fasting. In recent years, there seems to be quite a bit of information backing up that claim. In ancient times before obesity was a common issue and fasting was a way of life, there were significantly less heart disease and weight-related problems. A big part of this was because they lived solely on plant and meat based foods and there was natural fasting when food was not available. In recent times, however, it can be attributed as a benefit of fasting.

- Benefit Three: Helps with slowing down the aging process.
Another age-old claim to intermittent fasting is that it significantly slows down the process of aging. The science behind this claim is that fasting lowers the hormone IGF-1. This is the growth hormone that is often attributed too aging, tumor growth, and cancer risk. As people age, their intestinal stem cells begin to lose the ability to regenerate. These particular stem cells are the sources for all new intestinal cells. The age-related loss of stem cell function can simply be reversed with a twenty-four hour fast. On a recent study on mice, the researchers found that fasting dramatically increased the stem cells ability to impressively regenerate on both old and young mice. Mice and humans are quite similar anatomically so results are often the same. The cells begin breaking down fatty acids instead of glucose; this is a change that allows stem cells to become more regenerative. The slowing down of aging by allowing the stem cells to regenerate in mice has been so successful researchers are trying to come up with a medication that mimics the effects of fasting. The studies showed that not only did the stem cell regeneration slow down the aging process, it actually reversed it on a cellular level and significantly increased life longevity in the mice.

- Benefit Four: Sharper focus.

When your body is in a period of fasting, your body has to hyper-focus on the task at hand. This phenomenon occurs in a period of "starvation". It increases attention to detail and sharpens the mind. It makes sense when you think about when you eat a big meal. You generally feel sleepy and full afterward. This is where the term "food coma" comes from. You eat a big meal and want to take a nap. Intermittent fasting has the opposite effect. In a fast, your insulin is naturally low thereby giving you the ability to focus better on your task at hand. This is also the same reason that women on a ketogenic diet plan report that they have better focus and a clearer mind. The body is forced into a state of ketosis or fat burning, causing the brain to only focus on one thing at a time.

- Benefit five: Better cardiac health.

Better heart health is certainly a perk of engaging in the intermittent fasting lifestyle. The way it helps with cardiac health is that it lowers the risk factors for heart disease. Intermittent fasting aids in weight loss which helps to lower insulin and naturally regulate the body's other hormones. It can help to lower the blood pressure which can decrease the risk factors of heart attack and stroke. Intermittent fasting forces the body to burn its own fat stores which means less fat stored in the body which aids in lowered cholesterol and triglycerides. Fasting induces ketosis which helps to break down the fat stores and releases cholesterol destroying agents into the bloodstream. Better cardiac health was found in people that fasted just two days a week.

Intermittent Fasting and Cancer Patients

Intermittent fasting in cancer patients seems to have a promising future. There have been several studies done both on mice and on humans with good results. It seems that one benefit that intermittent fasting has on women is that it is helping to trigger the immune system.

The immune system in humans is designed to destroy and hunt down harmful pathogens in the body. When it comes to cancer though, the body seems to be not so good at finding and killing its own altered and abnormal cells, such as cancer cells. Many of the newer cancer treatments work on targeting the development and stimulation of the body's own immune system.

Now, recent research is finding that something as simple as a fasting lifestyle could be doing the work they have been trying to develop. There was a fairly new study at a university in California that was done on lab mice. This study mostly was surrounded around mesothelioma. This experiment used lab mice that had received chemotherapy along with a fasting diet and it showed that the immune system had a significantly easier time targeting and killing off breast cancer cells and skin cancer cells. The mice produced more cells that helped the immune system when on a fasting program; these cells included B cells and T cells. These cells actively target and destroy tumor cells. Along with that discovery, they learned that the cells that often protect tumors from chemotherapy which are called T regulatory cells were not found in the tumors following this protocol, which means that the chemotherapy drugs were able to do their job much better and with fewer barriers.

The same people that did this research on mice also did a piloted study with human cancer patients. This was mostly to learn if fasting programs with chemotherapy would be safe. The use of two-day fasts, four-day fasts, and water only fasts, along with calorie-restricted diets were all found to be safe and useful to cancer patients while being supervised by physicians. All the studies also showed that a fasting or intermittent fasting diet went along well with chemotherapy and could be useful in slowing the growth of tumors in cancer patients.

The side effects in cancer patients from chemotherapy were also affected in the studies. Side effects to chemotherapy can range from minor to crippling. Intermittent fasting can help to protect the body against side effects. One of the studies showed that a patient fasted for several days before the treatment and then ate normally right before their treatment. They did not appear to lose a dangerous amount of weight and it did not have any noticeable interference with their treatments. What did come out of it was significantly reduced side effects in the patients that were active in a fasting diet program. Patients that were part of the trial had less weakness and fatigue, less nausea, fewer headaches, and no vomiting at all. They also saw a reduced amount of dry mouth, cramps, mouth sores, and numbness.

The skeptics of the intermittent fasting lifestyle are concerned that it promotes eating patterns that are not healthy and could promote eating disorders. The research behind intermittent fasting in cancer patients does not support this, however. There have been several studies that show when guided by professionals, that it is safe for cancer fighters. There is minimal evidence that long-term calorie restriction could have the potential to have some negative effects, but most of these are not significant. For women who are battling cancer, it may be worth trying. The results appear to be safe and stable there seems to be a lot of hope with it for cancer patients. Be sure to only engage in intermittent fasting though, with the approval of your doctors and oncology teams.

Fasting and the Brain: The Effects It Has and Potentially Slowing Down Neurologic Diseases

Intermittent fasting is unsurprisingly good for the brain. There is a multitude of neurochemical changes that occur in the brain during a state of fasting. Neurotrophic factors are improved along with better cognitive function, resistance to stress, and reduction of inflammation. Intermittent fasting provides your brain with a challenge and the brain adapts to the test by creating and adapting pathways of stress response that allow your brain to better deal with disease and stress risks. The changes that happen during a period of fast mimic the chemical changes in the brain that happen with regular exercise. Both exercise and periods of fasting increase and better produce protein levels in the brain which helps to promote the growth of new and healthy neurons, and helps to improve the connection between the neurons and make the synapses stronger. Fasting can help to encourage and better produce new nerve cells that come from stem cells in the hippocampus. Fasting also helps to increase and stimulate the production of ketones by the liver, which neurons in the brain use as an energy source. Fasting helps to multiply the number of mitochondria in nerve cells as well since neurons are constantly adapting to stress by producing more mitochondria. Since mitochondria in the neurons are increased, the ability for new neurons to form and keep the connections between the neurons also is improved which ultimately leads to improving the abilities of memory and learning capabilities. Besides the impressive capabilities of intermittent fasting improving brain function, there is also evidence that intermittent has the ability to help enhance nerve cells to aid in the repair of DNA. The results of several studies showed that intermittent fasting helped to shift stem cells from a dormant state to self-renewal; because of this, it triggered the regeneration of organ systems based on stem cells. In conclusion, because of the mild stress fasting puts on the brain, it can help to slow down the growth of abnormal brain cells. By slowing those cells, it could potentially be slowing down or reversing the growth of cells that cause Alzheimer's and Parkinson's disease. The brain is an incredibly complex organ and it is a major breakthrough to show that something as simple as not eating for a few extra hours a day can possibly change and prevent devastating neurological diseases.

Chapter Two

What Is Hunger and How to Get Past the Feeling of It

Hunger is basically your body telling you it wants food and that you should feed it, or the desire or urge to eat. A big hurdle in intermittent fasting is overcoming the initial hunger that you feel. Basically, your mind is trying to convince you that you will die if you do not immediately eat. So it is important to convince your mind otherwise and break the cycle of immediately eating when you think you are hungry. The human body has evolved for thousands of years and is well equipped to handle significant periods of fasting. Training the mind, however, is the greater challenge. First, it is important to recognize that there are two main kinds of hunger. There is physical hunger, where your body is actually hungry and asking for food and there is psychological hunger, where your emotions are telling you they want food. It is essential to your success to be able to recognize the difference and the symptoms of physical versus psychological hunger.

Signs of physical hunger include hunger that comes on gradually and does not need to be satisfied immediately, it can be satisfied with any food, it causes satisfaction and no guilty emotions.

The signs of psychological hunger include sudden and urgent need to eat, often comes with specific cravings, leaves you feeling full to the point of discomfort, displeased with yourself, and guilt.

Getting through the hunger especially the phycological hunger in the middle of a fast can be a challenging mental obstacle. There are many good ways to try and help yourself get through the hunger. One of them is to be sure you are not mistaking hunger with dehydration.

106

Often, you think you are feeling pains of hunger when really your body simply wants water. Coffee and tea are excellent for helping to curb the feelings of hunger as well; sugar-free drinks are good options as well. Brushing your teeth has been proven to help reduce the hungry feelings as well. One of the best ways is to stay focused on something else and remain active. Doing something you enjoy or an activity where you are productive are easily the best hunger deterrents. It is easy for your time to fly right on by when you are engrossed in an activity and often before you know it, your fasting time has passed, anything to keep your mind engaged enough to break the craving or feelings of hunger.

Studies have shown that once your body adapts to fasting, the hormone ghrelin, which is the hormone that tells your body you what time you normally eat at, begins to adjust. Many women think that the longer you do not eat, or fast, the hungrier you become. This is false. Hunger comes and goes in a fast. After several days, your hormones begin to adjust. Many women say that the first four days are the most difficult with managing and adjusting to hunger. After about the fourth day, however, your hormones have significantly adjusted, and many have reported they become less and less hungry. Sometimes, when you are feeling hungry, it may actually be the ghrelin hormone telling you that you need salt. Sodium intake is quite important to the body. It has many critical functions in the human body. Salt is needed to help the heart function and pump adequately and is also key in cell-to-cell communication and is vital to helping the major organs function properly.

Getting through your first fast takes willpower and determination, but it does get easier. We are trained from an early age to be eating almost all the time to be healthy and lose weight. By engaging in intermittent fasting, you are retraining and conditioning your body to do something that it has forgotten it is meant to do. Fighting hunger is often the toughest battle for women who choose to endeavor on the tricky, yet beneficial route of intermittent fasting. There are also tools and techniques to help you overcome your hunger. Practicing meditation and yoga have shown to be significantly helpful in managing your feelings of hunger and recalibrating and clearing the mind. Essential oils have been shown to have positive effects on managing hunger and cravings as well. There are many tools available to help get a grip on controlling your hunger and feelings. Be sure to utilize some of them to help yourself get over this first hurdle.

How to Use Healthy Snacks to Help Adjust

Using healthy snacks is a good way to adjust to intermittent fasting. Gradually cutting out junk food and replacing them with foods that are healthy are an excellent way to prepare your body. If you are having trouble adjusting to a fasting period or are overeating when breaking a fast, using a healthy snack can really help. Make the last thing you eat before a fast be something high in good fat and low in carbs. Then make the first thing you eat after a fast be the same. You may need to gradually lengthen your fasts over time if you are just having too much trouble at first. Start with an eight hour fast and go from there. Reward yourself with a healthy snack after it. Healthy snacks are foods that are high in the good fats that will actually satisfy your hunger, not just mask it. Having a nutrient dense snack is what will satisfy the feeling best.

Examples of healthy snacks:

- Avocado
- Peanuts
- Soy nuts
- A spoonful of peanut butter
- Pumpkin or sunflower seeds

Hanger and Hanxiety

The hanger is real! Originally this term was meant as a joke to describe the progressive irritation of a hungry girl, it has now become an actual term used regularly. Hanger is a common term used to describe the irritable feeling that comes with being hungry. Many people that already deal with hanger issues may really struggle the first couple of days of fasting. As with most things, it will be easier to handle if you anticipate it and are prepared to handle it. If you know you get irritable while hungry, perhaps plan to do something that you find enjoyable to distract you. Take a walk, practice mindfulness, many have found meditation to be useful when going through a rough patch in the fasting. Keep in mind that it will pass. Your body will adjust after the first three days and it does get easier. Many women have said that the best way to combat their "hanger" is with laughter. Finding a funny picture, video, book or person significantly helped the feelings to pass! Also having herbal tea, coffee, or water can help with getting passed the irritability. The feelings of hanger are not pleasant to anyone so be sure you are ready with a potential distraction should the feeling occur.

The other hunger-induced feeling that can occur is anxiety or commonly referred to as 'hanxiety'. This is the uneasy or panicked feeling you have induced by hunger. It is essentially stress-induced anxiety. As with the angry, agitated feelings, it will pass. If you are prone to anxiety, be prepared with activities that you know will distract and relax you. Hunger induced anxiety is unpleasant and can be alarming. While not quite as common as a hanger, hunger-induced anxiety is a real feeling and should be treated appropriately. Many women have found that yoga, Pilates, or exercise can significantly help their anxiety as well as the earlier mentioned meditation, mindfulness exercises, headspace, essential oils and various other anxiety coping tools are helpful with getting through it. Just always remember that it is not permanent and you will adjust. If anxiety is a preexisting condition for you, it may be a good idea to consult with your doctor first and discuss ways to help you cope with the adjustment to minimize your anxiety and cause the least amount of stress on your mind and body systems.

Common Myths

As with any dieting or lifestyle change, there are always common myths and misconceptions that seem to accompany them. Debunking the common myths is important to better the understanding of the intermittent fasting concepts. When you first begin telling people what you are doing, in all likely hood someone will say that they have heard something bad about it. Since you have done your research, you know that the majority of the negative claims are in fact, false and that intermittent fasting is highly beneficial in a wide variety of ways. The most common myths are as follows: fasting is unnatural and unhealthy; it slows the metabolic rate; it causes loss of muscle tone; it can cause eating disorders and encourages overeating; and that you cannot exercise while fasting.

Myth One - Fasting Is Unnatural and Unhealthy for the Human Body

How false this myth is! Fasting is extremely natural. As stated before, in ancient and even stone age times, there were natural periods of fasting when meat could not be hunted, and berries and plants could not be gathered. This meant that people simply did not eat. Not only is intermittent fasting quite natural, but it is also even considered healthy. Humans are quite well adapted to long fasts because of the reasons above. This myth can certainly be debunked simply by history. Besides intermittent fasting being historically inaccurate, there are now studies and testimonies of the benefits of the intermittent fasting lifestyle.

Myth Two - Intermittent Fasting Slows Down the Metabolism

Intermittent fasting slowing down the metabolism is also an inaccurate claim. Intermittent fasting actually speeds up the metabolism because it naturally lowers the insulin and blood sugar. So really, intermittent fasting helps to regulate the hormones that affect your metabolism which is part of why it is so successful with weight loss.

Myth Three - Intermittent Fasting Causes Muscle Loss

Unless done incorrectly on a very thin person, intermittent fasting causing any significant muscle loss is unlikely. The event in which this could take place is if the body has no fat stores left and begins to eat muscle. This is highly unlikely though. Intermittent fasting does not cause serious muscle loss or breakdown when used correctly. There is some controversy that doing too much cardio while fasting can cause some minor breakdown of muscle tissues, but there are little science and research to back these claims. While anytime there is weight loss, there is generally some mild degree of muscle loss, though it is easily built back up with proper supplements and exercise.

Myth Four - Intermittent Fasting Causes Eating Disorders

If you have already struggled with anorexia or bulimia, fasting may not be for you. While it certainly does not cause eating disorders, you do not want to fall in too poor diet habits on accident. If you have a history of an eating disorder, talk to your doctor or therapist about the healthiest way to proceed with the intermittent fasting program. Planning and cooking meals and snacks ahead of time may be quite helpful with this, same with having a meal and eating plan that you stick too is helpful. Having a strong support system is especially important if you have previously overcome an eating disorder. Though as stated above, intermittent fasting does not cause eating disorders.

Myth Five - Intermittent Fasting Encourages Overeating

If you break your fast correctly and stick to simple rules, overeating should not typically occur. Intermittent fasting actually shrinks down the stomach which theoretically leaves the body craving less food. Especially if you break your fast with a food high in good fat, then it breaks down fat first which leaves you feeling more satisfied. The majority of all overeating is typically psychological. The other reason that this is false is that because intermittent fasting naturally lowers the blood sugar and insulin levels, it leaves you feeling less hungry because of the stability in the blood sugars. While the first few days can be rough, ultimately you should crave much less food. While your body is in the adjustment period, this is generally when the most overeating occurs. Typically, after adjusting to a more constricted stomach, people often feel uncomfortably full once they begin eating after a fast and do not want to have large meals or eat too much.

Myth Six - You Cannot Exercise While in a Fast

Not being able to exercise while in a fast is another common misconception. Many people fast all night and through midday if they are on a sixteen-hour fast, eight-hour feeding schedule. A fair amount of research states that doing your exercise first thing in the morning is the ideal time to work out, and this technically puts you in the middle of your fast. Many women actually work out in replace of breakfast. They have reported that working out first thing in the morning helps them wake up and prepare them for the day far more adequately than their previous morning habits. Since fasting does not necessarily alter your diet, just when you eat, your workout habits should not need to be drastically adjusted. The only time when you may want to go easy on working out is when you are first adjusting either to intermittent fasting itself or adjusting to a ketogenic diet. In these cases, it is recommended to rest and allow the adjustment period, as to help with avoiding keto flu symptoms and overstressing of the body systems.

Once you are appropriately adjusted, however, exercise will aid in weight loss and an overall healthier diet. The one string of truth to this myth is that it may be unwise to do exceptionally intense workouts while in a fast. There are chances you may get some muscle breakdown if the intensity is too high for a fasted work out.

Common Mistakes

With every diet or lifestyle change, there are common mistakes that can alter your potential success. Intermittent fasting is not a clear or precise art; there are many variables that can affect your results. There are, however, simple mistakes that can damage your results that are quite easily preventable. Many do not even realize they are making them. Being aware of your habits is very important to success with intermittent fasting. Like with any lifestyle change, adjustment takes time, and nobody gets it right all at once.

Not Eating Enough in the Feeding Period

Not getting enough to eat after a fast is a common mistake. The stomach has a certain amount of dispensability. Meaning it can shrink and expand to a certain amount. While in a fast, it contracts and adapts to handling less. When you are eating a lot, it expands and gets used to accommodate larger amounts of food. When you are preparing to break your fast, you naturally want to eat heavy foods that are very dense. This is a common mistake because, with your stomach in a shrunken state, you quickly do not have room for the good things like vegetables and fibers. It is important to get enough foods with good fats, especially at the beginning of breaking your fast. Breaking your fast with good fats such as avocado, eggs, peanut butter is a good way to kick start your appetite and to transition the body from a self-fat burning state to burning the fats that you feed it. Maintaining enough calories is important too. When you do not get enough calories, the effects are more undesirable and detrimental. Meal planning and research can really help with this as well as planning when the best time of day to break your fast is.

Coffee and Tea Creamers

This is another common mistake that people unintentionally do that causes a break in fast without realizing it. Even a half-tablespoon of coffee creamer or almond milk is enough to trigger an insulin response and break a fast. As soon as you include the substance in your beverage, you may as well end the fast because you will need to start over. Adjusting to coffee in black can be difficult if it is not what you are accustomed to. Many people that cannot seem to get used to it simply switch to herbal teas.

Not Drinking Enough Water

Another common mistake is simply not keeping yourself hydrated enough. Many times, when you feel like you may be hungry, it may actually be your body telling you to hydrate it. Women were shocked to find that many hunger pains during a fast were curbed by simply drinking water or tea. The body also demands more salt on an intermittent fasting diet. Be sure to get enough water and salt as these are essential to getting good, healthy results. Drinking enough water and staying well hydrated also helps to prevent and get over the keto flu, if you are also following the ketogenic diet. Hydration is key to any change in diet and will nearly always improve your results.

Not Having Enough Support

Often times with any diet this is the biggest cause of failure. Support for a life change is absolutely a necessity. Without having a support system to lean on, ask questions and discuss ideas with, most people are not successful. If you are struggling and frustrated, be sure to find someone who is also going through the changes and adjustments that come with changing your habits to an intermittent fasting lifestyle.

There are many online support groups with great support systems and knowledge to share. Changing your life is hard as it is and it is nearly impossible to do alone.

The Myth of Breakfast — Is It Really the Most Important Meal of the Day?

From a young age, it has been drilled into our heads that breakfast is the most important meal of the day; however, the more research that comes out regarding intermittent fasting is beginning to tell us that breakfast may not be as beneficial and necessary as we are programmed to think. Over time, it has been proven that there is no real negative effect or significance to skipping breakfast. The pesky little hormone of ghrelin is partially responsible for putting us in the habit of eating breakfast every morning. This is the hormone that tells us to eat at the same time every day. Part of why we feel we need to eat breakfast is that it is simply a habit ingrained in our brains and in our hormones for most of our lives.

Individuals have recently found that once they adapted and retrained their bodies to not be expecting to be fed first thing in the morning, that there were actually little to no negative effects in their daily lives and routines. To put it in simple terms, our bodies naturally fast overnight, eating breakfast is breaking the fast first thing in the morning and it is not necessarily at a benefit. Individuals who skipped breakfast were also shown to have burned more calories during the day as opposed to those that ate breakfast in the morning. In the morning, as we have theoretically fasted overnight unless you are a sleepwalking eater, you are already in or near a mild state of ketosis, as your blood glucose stores have been depleted overnight. Within several hours of waking up, our body hormones will adopt that will make it stronger in the long run. The growth hormone gets released and this will help improve insulin sensitivity.

Insulin sensitivity is important to maintaining a fast comfortably and is the hormone responsible for telling you that your body wants to be fed. Staying as sensitive as possible to insulin helps to keep the blood glucose levels stable which helps you to feel less hungry and avoid overeating. If you decide skipping breakfast is not an option and you are unwilling to give it a try, it will be necessary to arrange your fasting around breakfast. However, the worst type of breakfast you can have is a high carbohydrate, sugary breakfast after breaking a fast. This throws the hormones out of balance by raising your blood glucose and causing the insulin response. It will not only completely end ketosis but will make it very difficult to reestablish it for several days. So, the bottom line is if you do not think you can skip breakfast, at the very least avoid an unhealthy one.

Many people want breakfast simply out of a lifetime of habit and breaking that routine is quite difficult at first. Many women find that working out first thing in the morning is a great way to get past the breakfast cravings. Working out in the morning is a great time to get in some exercise and wake you up for the day

Our Bodies Already Feed Us in the Morning

Ultimately, our bodies already are feeding us in the morning because you should be in a fat burning state. Once you are in a state of fat burning, it is unnecessary to eat breakfast because your body is already burning its reserved fat cell. When you wake up in the morning, you are already in a state of mild ketosis, or in the fat burning state. Eating breakfast breaks the ketosis and you go back to converting carbs for energy. Most women reported that once they adjusted to not eating breakfast in the morning, they hardly noticed a difference. The beauty of ketosis is that your blood sugar is stable and your insulin is low. This means that your body should not be giving off the feelings of hunger. With lowered insulin, the hormone ghrelin is also low and will not tell your brain that it needs to be fed first thing in the morning.

Usually, after a short adjustment period, many women neither crave or need to eat breakfast.

How Intermittent Fasting Can Slow Down Aging Process

One great benefit to intermittent fasting is that it can actually slow down the aging process. Mitochondria are structures in the cells that produce energy. They change in their shape in the response of energy demand. However, as we age, they lose the ability to do so. In a study that focused on mitochondria in the cells, there was evidence that they were able to retain 'youthfulness' longer by dietary restrictions such as intermittent fasting.

Chapter Three

The Lean Gain Method

Often, when people hear of the term "intermittent fasting" they also think if the term "lean gains." Lean gains are one of the programs that brought intermittent fasting to light in more recent years. Originally designed for rapid muscle building and fat loss, it has become a popular term in the dieting industry.

Lean gains is a dieting approach that basically takes three types of dieting and melts them all into one. The lean gain approach was created as an optimal solution to getting fit and having an efficient healthy diet. Basically, the lean gain method consists of intermittent fasting, usually the sixteen hours fast and the eight-hour feeding window; however, there is some debate on whether or not women benefit more from a fourteen hour fast with a ten-hour eating window. There is some variation depending on personal preference and need. It consists of weight training, classic lifts and squats, and all the typical strength training techniques.

Lean gains also consist of high protein diet on a daily basis while strength training days are high on carbs and low fat; nevertheless, the rest of the time is on moderate fat and low carbs. The lean gain approach is one that many people have heard of and associate with the term intermittent fasting. It was ultimately designed to help men get fit and ripped fast while using intermittent fasting as an aid and timed meals and calorie intake. In the lean gain method, it is recommended that you eat post workout or strength training. It is also recommended to perform strength training three times per week and there have been some decent results with the studies. Many subjects lost a significant amount of body fat while gaining significant muscle. Essentially, the lean gain approach tricks your body into thinking it is on a diet, while really you are just limiting the time that you are feeding and adjusting your caloric, fat, and carb intakes.

The lean gain method is one of the names that brought intermittent fasting to light and made it popular in recent culture. Like with all things that have to do with intermittent fasting, it is beneficial to many but not necessarily right for everyone. While women can certainly participate and have good results from the lean gains system and protocols, it was and always will be more targeted for men interested in strength training and fast results.

Most women engage in intermittent fasting by following one of two of the most popular protocols. There is the 'sixteen eight protocol'. The sixteen eight protocol is where you fast for sixteen hours and then have an eight hour feeding period. This is popular as it can be a way of life.

Getting Started With Intermittent Fasting

Most Common Fast Periods:

- Sixteen hours fast with an eight-hour feeding window
- Twelve and twelve-twelve hour fast, twelve-hour feeding window
- Fourteen and ten-fourteen hour fast, ten hour feeding period
- The twenty-four hour fast should be performed no more than two times per week

When jumping into the lifestyle of intermittent fasting, first establish a plan. Do your research and decide what fast is best for you. There will be a certain amount of trial and error. A good place to start is the sixteen hour fast with an eight-hour feeding window. Plan out what you are going to break your fast with ahead of time and have a time planned. It is best to do it on a day when you are busy and have plans, especially if you tend to be an emotional eater. Keeping busy will help with keeping you distracted and absent-mindedly eating. Have a stock of herbal teas and black coffee if you think you are going to have trouble your first day. Keep it in mind that it will get easier. It takes a few days for your body to adjust to the fasting lifestyle. But remember, it will adjust. Our bodies are well equipped for prolonged periods of fasting, it is just an adjustment period. It is also okay to not be successful immediately. There will be a trial and error and the standard fasting periods do not always work for everyone. It is okay to adjust your schedule to what better fits your needs, your lifestyle, your workout schedule, and your daily life in general. It is ok to adjust your fast and eating period as well.

While the sixteen and eight-fast and feeding period is easily the most common and can be safely used every day, it does not mean it is necessarily the best fit for you personally. If you start off with a sixteen-hour fast and find it is simply too much for you at first, start with a smaller window. Start with a twelve-hour fast and build up to where you want to be. Some women do better with a fourteen-hour fast and a ten-hour feeding window, and then some prefer a twenty-hour fast and a four-hour feeding window. Everyone is different and what is most important is what works for your schedule, lifestyle, comfort levels, and that ultimately gives you the best results with fasting.

Planning Your Meals After a Fast

Planning your post fast meals has a lot of room for customization. Finding the best solution for you can require some trial and error. Once you break your fast, it is important not to immediately inhale your food and continue eating nonstop through your fasting period. Eat something that is high in good fat and go from there. Many women find that in their feeding period they only eat two regular meals, while others eat three. Some prefer to just snack continuously through the feeding period. While you are still adjusting to intermittent fasting, it is not uncommon to feel ravenously hungry at first. This is part of why it is so important to break your fast slowly and with certain foods. When first getting started, one of the absolute most important tricks to success is having your day and meals planned out and then sticking to them. The more you have planned, the less likely you will be tempted with foods that do not go well with intermittent fasting. As with any diet change, you will be more successful with self-monitoring. Having a plan helps you to keep self-control better and you will be less likely to binge eat or impulse eat after coming out of your fasting state. When you are first adjusting is when this is most critical. You will be very hungry at first because it takes three to five days for your hormones to self-regulate. Once your insulin has naturally stabilized, ghrelin hormone will also adjust and begin telling you that you are hungry at your new meal times. The body likes routine and adjusting to fasting is simply teaching your body a new routine. Planning your meals and knowing what and when you are going to eat will drastically help with the adjustment period.

Breaking Your Fast

Care should be taken when breaking your fast, so you do not overwhelm your digestive system. It is important to not overeat right after you have completed your fast as this is a critical time for your digestive system. While in a fast, your metabolism is in a state of hormonal and physiological adaptions so in order to not disrupt and irritate the digestive tract, it is essential to follow some basic guidelines for ending your fast and entering your period of feeding time.

Guidelines While Breaking Your Fast

First, finding something to stimulate the digestive tract without releases insulin is ideal. Making a drink with lemon water, sea salt, two tablespoons of apple cider vinegar and cinnamon is a great way to wake up your digestive tract without upping your insulin, just hot lean water works as well. The citric acid from lemons helps to give the digestive enzymes a bit of a boost. The broth is another good fast breaker, especially bone broth. Bone broth is great for boosting collagen and easing your digestive tract back in. These starter beverages are especially useful for breaking a long fast; more than twenty hours when your gut is "asleep." For breaking a routine, twelve to sixteen-hour fast foods high in good fats are good for that. Avocados, a few eggs, or fish are all suitable for breaking a fast. The body will be in low-level ketosis and it will be more beneficial for it to transfer from burning its own fat to burning an ingested fat as opposed to a more complex carb to break down. When breaking a fast, the first meal should be relatively small. Under five hundred calories is ideal. This will help to re-acclimate your digestive system and adjust to food again.

The other common style of intermittent fasting is the twenty-four-hour protocol. This is where you do not eat for twenty-four hours. However, this protocol is slightly riskier, and you should not engage in it more than two days a week. When first beginning to fast, it is important to be mentally prepared for the challenge. At first, it will not come easily, and you will be fighting hunger. Essentially you are retraining your body that you do not need food as often as it thinks you do and this can take time.

The Four Main Types of Fasting

There are really four main types of fasting with different benefits. The most popular is intermittent fasting where you only eat for certain parts of the day. In a biological sense, all fasting is intermittent because you cannot simply live without calories and food. Fasting is more of a lifestyle approach and is certainly better for body composition.

The four types of fasting are intermittent fasting, prolonged fasting, liquid fasting, and dry fasting.

- Intermittent Fasting

Intermittent fasting is essentially what has been discussed this whole guide. Only feeding for certain parts of the day. As mentioned throughout, it has many benefits, the most popular being weight loss.

- Prolonged Fasting

There is also a form of fasting called prolonged fasting. This is a fast that lasts twenty-four to seventy-two hours. This is really only safe to do one to two times a month. It is good for cell rejuvenation. It is good to do on occasion as the body goes and hunts out the old and dying cells and feeds on them. This is called autophagy. Autophagy is basically how your body recycles cells. Prolonged fasting is good for longevity and fat burning. However, once you pass the forty-eight hours mark, there begins to have a few negative effects. So, if you choose to partake in a prolonged fast, twenty-four to forty-eight hours is the sweet spot. While this fast has its benefits, be sure to carefully monitor yourself throughout, and be sure to only follow this fasting protocol one to two times per month as using a prolonged fast too often, will create a calorie deficiency.

- The Liquid Fast

Metabolically speaking, the liquid fast is not a true fast. However, it is good for your digestive system. The liquid fast protocol is consisting of all liquids, and it is good to do one to two times a week. Liquid fasting is a good way to give the digestive system a break. Liquids are much easier to digest than solid foods. The liquid fast can consist of just about any liquid, jello type products, tea, and coffee. If you have a sensitive digestive system or irritable bowel, the liquid fast can be beneficial especially.

- The Dry-Fast

The dry fast is a rather extreme fast. To dry fast means to ingest nothing — no food and no water for an extended period of time, usually twenty-four hours. This fast is generally quite extreme and should only be done every three to six months. There are two different types of dry fasts. The soft fast, which is where you can still brush your teeth and the hard fast is where you do not. The dry fast does come with some risks; however, there are also benefits. It is extreme though and should only be done a few times a year. The dry fast is good if you have a lot of inflammation in your body. The lack of fluids pulls the water from the area that is inflamed. The dry fast is a good way to restart your digestive system and help your body to rid of retained water and extra edema. It should be used with great caution and great infrequency, however.

Getting It Right for You

Keep in mind that when you begin intermittent fasting, it is more of a lifestyle change than an actual diet and it is okay to not get it right a first. Finding out what works for you is a major part of being successful with intermittent fasting. Many women have found different schedules that work best for them. The other key point to keep in mind, is what is the rush? You do not need to figure out what best works for you on the first day. It is a good idea to take a little time and figure out what works best for you and your lifestyle before getting started. Find meal recipes and plan what you will eat ahead of time if you are unsure of things and feel you do not have enough support, try and find a friend to do it with. There are numerous online resources that offer great ideas, support, and advice. It is helpful to talk to your family doctor or a nutritionist before starting. They can potentially help you to tailor your diet and schedule to a system of eating and fasting that works for you the most adequately.

It is certainly a learning curve to adjust to such a lifestyle and it is important to cut yourself some slack. Try not to get frustrated if you see friends or other people have more success or different effects than you are having at first. Every woman is different, and every metabolism is different as well. It is always okay to give yourself time both to adjust and figure out your ideal program. A healthy lifestyle is not built in a day and there will be setbacks and annoyances along the way. One of the most important things to remember is that no matter how long it takes, or how difficult it is for you to adjust, you are still doing laps around the people that are not trying!

Special Advice for Overweight Women and Intermittent Fasting

Many people are drawn to intermittent fasting because of the weight loss benefits. While intermittent fasting is helpful and beneficial for weight loss, it is important to follow the correct protocols while starting out. Intermittent fasting is very beneficial for weight loss and one of the main reason women are interested in the lifestyle to start with. If you are overweight and want to participate in intermittent fasting for weight loss, it is best to thoroughly discuss with your doctor first. While some form of fasting can be beneficial to everyone, not all types or styles are right for every person. Discuss with your doctor your goals and what they believe the healthiest way to do it is.

Generally, overcoming hunger and emotional eating are the biggest hurdles. Many people are overweight because they tend to eat their feelings and emotions. Often, weight loss is difficult because women tend to turn to food for comfort. Intermittent fasting for weight loss does extremely well with a ketogenic type of diet. Combining the two gives excellent and fairly quick results. The other thing you will want to do if you are overweight and want to give intermittent fasting a try is to begin some form of exercise routine. This can start out as simply walking around the block or going for a bike ride. Doing some form of work out will help to allow fat to be burned more efficiently and will likely speed up the weight loss process. Many women see rapid weight loss when starting the intermittent fasting program while others see fewer results until combined with another traditional diet. Intermittent fasting has been so popular in the last few years because it has been so helpful to women losing weight.

Bypass or Weight Loss Surgery and Intermittent Fasting

It appears that there is a bit of controversy when it comes to whether or not intermittent fasting is a good idea after having weight loss surgery. Weight loss surgery is typically a gastric bypass; when the stomach is cut down to a small pocket and removed; a gastric sleeve where the stomach is contained to the approximate size of a banana or the lap band surgery where a band is placed around the stomach to make it smaller in size. Women that have had weight loss surgery have typically exhausted all diet options and needed the surgery to help them to lose the weight. Adding intermittent fasting in after a weight loss surgery can be tricky. Since the size of the stomach has been significantly reduced, calories and nutrients are not as easily absorbed. Since the intermittent fasting diet is meant to be over a feeding period, this often does not go well with bariatric surgery patients because they cannot physically eat enough calories to be healthy over the feeding period. If you are really interested in intermittent fasting after a weight loss surgery, then it is best to discuss with you

Type Two Diabetes

There are some recent studies that imply that intermittent fasting can be beneficial to individuals with type two diabetes. Fasting and diabetes have had a bit of controversy surrounding it but with some recent and updated information, there is some evidence that it can help regulate insulin and blood glucose levels. As mentioned above, intermittent fasting aids and allows the body hormones, like blood glucose and insulin, to naturally lower and regulate. Fasting for insulin regulation appeared to be especially helpful for women that have had trouble maintaining a diabetic diet seven days a week. It was suggested that if fasted for two twenty-four-hour periods in a week, that insulin and blood sugar levels stabilized in the diabetic patient. This new evidence can really help to improve the lives of diabetics everywhere. Regardless of the research, it is still best to consult with your regular doctor before using intermittent fasting as a diabetic.

Age

It appears that once you are over the age of eighteen, there are little negative effects of intermittent fasting in any healthy adult. In ancient times, intermittent fasting was practiced by all ages and they all seemed to benefit from the lifestyle. Granted, the times were different and they had little choice other than to fast due to having to hunt and gather food. There is very limited evidence that says age matters or is of significance to any healthy adult that wants to participate in intermittent fasting.

Children and Intermittent Fasting

There is a bit of medical controversy over whether children should participate in the intermittent fast. Most doctors agree that they should if the child is overweight or obese. Intermittent fasting can be very beneficial for weight loss in kids and teenagers. It can be a particularly hard adjustment, however. Kids tend to like to snack all day long and this can be difficult to break. It is important that the meals the child consumes are very nutrient dense and satisfying. Start with three meals a day in a twelve-hour window and then gradually attempt to bring it down to two meals a day. As long as the meals are heavy in good nutrients and good fats, most kids adapt with little trouble. Intermittent fasting is great for overweight kids and teens as well as athletic teens that are trying to build more muscle.

The negativity surrounding intermittent fasting in children mostly comes from a presumption that not eating will stunt growth. There is no scientific evidence that supports this claim and intermittent fasting is not typically recommended in small or young children anyway. Most research says that if the kid is overweight or trying to build muscle for sports, it is acceptable.

Long-Term and Negative Effects

There is little official research on long-term fasting effects, but what there is research on, shows that there are very few negative long-term effects on the body systems from intermittent fasting. Like the people who lived in stone ages and ancient times, fasting is normal, and our bodies are well equipped to handle it. However, it is important to remember that humans have not been cavemen for hundreds of years so it does take some adapting. While the majority of intermittent fasting has good health benefits, there are some negative effects that can occur. As with any diet or lifestyle change, it is important to be aware of all effects.

Feeling Full to the Point of Discomfort

This can occur when you have been fasting for a while. Your body gets used to having a reduced stomach size and when you first eat, you have to readjust to the amount of food you intake. With intermittent fasting, depending on your feeding window, you generally have to get some large dense meals to get the appropriate number of calories to be healthy especially right before you head into a fast. Getting used to having a full stomach for a few hours is simply something you will have to adjust too, to keep up the intermittent fasting program. The other unfortunate part of having to eat large nutrient dense meals is that it can add stress to your body and digestive systems.

Reliance on Caffeine

Another less than positive long-term effect is that you tend to get over addicted to caffeine. Mainly tea and coffee. Since coffee and tea are allowed, many women drink an abundance of it during a fast to stay energized. Unfortunately, a caffeine addiction comes with its own issues. This side effects can include anxiety, sleep deprivation, mood swings, and weight gain. For the average everyday caffeine addict, these side effects can eventually be problematic.

Athletic Performance Can Suffer

While it is generally good and effective to work out during a fast, you should not do extremely intense workouts, which means sometimes your athleticism can suffer. If you are on the two days a week for a twenty-four-hour schedule, you can still do heavy and intense weight training. There are studies that show without careful regulation, performance does eventually begin to suffer especially with cardio type exercise such as performance running.

Heartburn

Heartburn is a common occurrence during intermittent fasting, especially when first adjusting to the schedule and lifestyle. It often does eventually go away after five or six weeks but not always. The reason that heartburn occurs is that the body is confused by the abnormal eating pattern and lets off acid in the stomach periodically. When you suddenly change your eating pattern, the stomach tries to keep it on the schedule that it was on. Some people adjust quickly and some simply never adjust and have to deal with the heartburn. If it does persist, you can see your doctor, and antacids often help.

Headaches Throughout the Fast

Many people complain of headaches while fasting. There is some speculation about what causes them. Some say it is being in the state of ketosis, while others say it is simply dehydration and should go away with water intake. Likely, it is either or both that causes the head pain many people get every time they fast, unfortunately. You can play around with water intake and the amount of time you fast to try and ease some of the headaches.

Reoccurring Diarrhea

This is a surprisingly frequent occurrence with intermittent fasting. Many women get diarrhea of varying degrees while in a fast. This is typically due to the high fluid intake; a large amount of coffee, water, and tea. Often women have complained that the longer the fast, the more explosive the diarrhea is. Often it can be controlled with over the counter medications, but is an unpleasant side effect, regardless.

Long-Term Effects

Unfortunately, there is very limited research on the long-term effects of intermittent fasting on the body systems. There is evidence of increased lifespan and decreased aging, but the studies remain limited. Very few people stay in the intermittent lifestyle program for years on end. Historically, it was helpful and had great benefits for the people alive in the stone ages. In modern times, however, there simply is not enough research to back up the claims of zero negative long-term effects. This does not mean though that the potential negative effects of intermittent fasting actually exist. Overall, intermittent fasting is fairly safe to do for extended periods of time and gives many people great results for a variety of things.

Chapter Four

Evaluate Your Progress

Finding what works best for you is one of the biggest challenges when engaging in intermittent fasting. Intermittent fasting is about the time period you are eating in as opposed to what exactly you are eating. Even with that being said, it is important that you find eating habits that are suitable for your needs. Planning ahead when you are intermittent fasting is probably the most important piece of advice to help with success. Consider your habits and daily patterns and try to figure out ways to break up your bad habits. Do you like to get fast food on your way home? Try and plan ahead with a meal in the car. You will be surprised to see how quickly you can break a bad eating habit if you get out in front of it.

Finding Your Suitable Eating Portion

Portion control also plays an important role in the intermittent fasting way of life. It is important to monitor your portion size, especially when breaking a fast. While you are in a fasting state, your stomach constricts. When you begin to eat again, your stomach expands. If you do not manage your portion sizes when breaking a fast, your stomach will expand swiftly and your body will spend much more of your feeding period trying to insist it needs more food because your stomach has expanded.

Is Intermittent Fasting for You?

Before you jump headlong into the lifestyle of intermittent fasting, make sure that it is the proper choice for you personally. It is not a bad idea to consult with a doctor, nutritionist or dietician before beginning. Certain health risk factors make the intermittent fasting protocols unhealthy for certain individuals. While most women can certainly benefit, there are always exceptions and it is important to be a good fit for the diet to maintain good long-term health. Generally speaking, intermittent has health benefits that can be good for nearly everyone. There are certain situations that require you to proceed with caution when considering this type of eating pattern including pregnancy and nursing mothers, bariatric surgery patients, recovering from an eating disorder, and several other situations that should be approached with caution.

When to Stop Intermittent Fasting

Examples:

- Uncontrolled binge eating
- Metabolic disruption
- Lost menstrual cycles
- Early onset menopause
- Eating disorder relapse

There may be a time when you are engaging in the lifestyle of intermittent fasting that the protocols are no longer healthy for your lifestyle, body chemistry, mental health, or physical health. While it can be beneficial to most women, if you are finding you cannot control your binge eating, no matter what technique you try, it may be better to shorten your fasts. If you find your menstrual periods have become abnormal, your mood is too out of whack, or something simply just does not feel right, stop the lifestyle immediately. You do not want to do something that can permanently harm your health.

It is okay to take a step back and evaluate your goals and where you are in life. Not every dietary change is right for every woman and that is okay. You will know what diet plan is right for you, and if you really enjoy the benefits and lifestyle of intermittent fasting, you can talk to a doctor or nutritionist to determine which is the best and the safest way to proceed with intermittent fasting. There are cases where intermittent fasting simply is not right for. Knowing yourself and your body well enough to determine what feels right and what works best for you is important to any diet change or lifestyle. As was mentioned previously, it is okay to not get it right at first.

Pregnancy and Fasting

Pregnancy and fasting is a bit of uncharted territory when it comes down to it. Many doctors say to not do it, that it is not safe and that you really should be consuming an extra three to five hundred calories per day while other doctors say it is not such a big deal. The best advice that can ultimately be given on the subject is if you choose to continue intermittent fasting while pregnant, proceed with utmost caution.

If you are determined to continue the intermittent lifestyle during your pregnancy, consider a slightly easier schedule. Try and fourteen and ten-hour fast, or a twelve and twelve schedule. It is very important to get adequate nutrition throughout the pregnancy and to consume foods that are high in fiber. During the third trimester, it is often necessary to bump up your calorie intake a little to ensure you and the fetus are getting adequate nutrition the remainder of the pregnancy. If you are unsure if you should continue intermittent fasting or do not feel comfortable with it, it is wise to consult with a trusted family physician or your OBGYN to see what they think is safe for you and the fetus.

Breastfeeding is also uncharted territory when it comes down to intermittent fasting. Generally, it is discouraged because it can affect your milk production which could potentially harm your baby and slow the growth and progression. Overall it is best to avoid intermittent fasting while pregnant and nursing unless under very careful monitoring by a doctor.

Polycystic Ovarian Syndrome and Intermittent Fasting

Polycystic ovaries are a fairly common disease in women. This disease causes a hormone shift and can have any undesirable effects on women. Many women struggle with weight gain and difficulty losing weight as a side effect of the disease. While there are not very many studies about how intermittent fasting affects the disease, there is evidence that combining intermittent fasting with a keto diet significantly helped to regulate the hormones and made weight loss possible for polycystic ovarian syndrome patients. There does seem to be some potential hope with using intermittent fasting to help treat and maintain diseases like polycystic ovarian syndrome and other hormonal disorders. Time and additional research will tell us if intermittent fasting has a future in helping with this disease.

Overcoming Binging

A struggle many women live and fight with is binge eating. Binge eating is to eat an excessive amount, even though your body is no longer hungry, and it is generally a psychological habit. Binge eating actually is considered an eating disorder now. Binge eating is especially difficult for women that tend to be emotional eaters. Many women turn to food to control their feeling and this is both common and can be quite a challenge to overcome.

Emotional eating is when you literally want to eat whenever you have a strong feeling about something. Emotionally eating, or eating your feeling as some call it, very easily leads to binge eating. As with any bad habit, binge eating falls into the category of learning to break the habit. This is naturally much easier said than done. Many women have found distraction techniques as helpful to get control of their binge eating. Yoga, Pilates, and meditation are great ways to clear your mind and pull your focus away from emotionally eating.

Overcoming binging can be a real challenge and can take real work and willpower. It also is not always necessarily able to be broken immediately. It is important that you learn to listen to what your body is telling you instead of your emotions and this will help with overcoming binge eating. Many women need a professional psychologist or counselor to get over binge eating. Eating can also be an addiction and sometimes, advanced help is needed to break the unhealthy cycle of overeating. If you realize you are out of control with your binge eating, do not hesitate to get help, there are many good resources for support for women.

Adjusting Your Intermittent Fasting Schedule

Where there is intermittent fasting, there is also an adjustment period. The nice thing about intermittent fasting is that the schedule is determined by what works for you and your schedule. While the flexibility is convenient, it is still an adjustment for your body, for your mind, and your day to day activities. You will need to be cautious and really listen to what your body is telling you when you are starting out with intermittent fasting. Just because the sixteen hours fast with the eight-hour feeding window is popular, it does not mean it cannot be adjusted to fit your needs. Many women do better with a fourteen-hour fast and a ten-hour feeding window, however, sixteen is simply too much for them. This is the beauty of the fasting schedule; it is flexible and can be adjusted to your individual needs.

Chapter Five

How to Get the Best Out of Intermittent Fasting

Combining Intermittent Fasting with Exercise

Combining intermittent fasting with exercise is one of the best ways to get the most benefits and best results out of intermittent fasting. Combining work out with intermittent fasting and any other diet; like ketogenic, paleo or any other low carb type program will give you the best and the quickest results for weight loss. There are many ways to exercise including cardio, strength training or lifting, yoga, and Pilates. Any of these exercise styles and regiments can be beneficial and help with your ultimate goal of weight loss and a healthier life, but certain workouts have certain benefits. There are also time frames to exercise in during a fast that will help to optimize your results. Cardio is ideal for fat burning and strength training for building muscle. Yoga is great for core strength and certain yoga poses can actually help to regulate certain hormones. Nearly all exercise has benefits if you can find the time and the drive to make it part of your daily lifestyle.

When to Work Out

Most would consider the opportune time to work out to be in the middle of a fast. For example, let's say you started your fast at ten at night, working out after you wake up in the morning is considering an ideal time to work out or exercise as it is in the middle of your fast. You should still have ample energy as your body will not be expecting to be fed until later. Working out in the morning is also a great way to get going in the morning and is a natural way of waking up. Doing your work out in the middle or beginning of your fast is usually superior and you will feel better with better results as opposed to doing your work out toward the end of your fast.

136

When you are nearing the end of your fasting period, your body tends to be more fatigued and depleted of energy and you may find your work out less satisfying and beneficial. Some women choose to do their work out during their feeding period. This is generally not quite as beneficial as working out during the fast itself but is still better than not working out at all. Besides working out for strength, weight loss and overall health, exercise is proven to release mood-improving endorphins and boost energy. Overall, it is ideal to workout midway through your fast, but as mentioned, if you cannot work out mid fast or if your schedule does not allow it, anytime you can fit it in is better than not at all. Working out is quite important to help achieve the best possible results, so it is better to fit it in where you can than not at all!

Yoga and Pilates to Aid in Hormonal Balance

Many people have heard of the wonderful benefits of practicing yoga and Pilates. Yoga is relaxing, great for flexibility, and improving core and body strength. Yoga has been known to aid in pain relief and improve the mood, reset the mind and help with focus. Yoga is a great natural way to give your body a boost and to help relax and de-stress. Basically, yoga brings the three main elements together; exercise, breathing, and meditation. Pilates has a similar effect except it tends to focus more on lengthening and strengthening all the major and large muscle groups. Pilates particularly improves strength, body awareness, and balance. What is less known about Pilates and yoga is that it can actually help to stabilize and regulate the body's hormones with certain poses. The yoga poses can subtly pressurize and depressurize certain glands of the body. These minor compressions and decompressions can help to regulate hormonal secretions. Therefore, certain yoga poses can help to balance and stimulate certain endocrine functions. Many common negative feelings can be attributed to a hormonal imbalance. Feelings like being constantly tired, low self-esteem, anxiety, and emotional eating with a slow metabolism can all possible be effects of a hormonal imbalance in women.

A few of even the most basic yoga poses can help with hormone regulation. An easy pose that can have a big effect is the 'rabbit pose' also known as the Sasangasana pose. This is a beginner pose that nearly anyone can do that works to stimulate the thyroid gland. The thyroid gland is on your neck and is a horn responsible for secreting growth regulating hormones and metabolic function. To get into this yoga pose, start by sitting on your heels in 'hero pose' (sitting on your legs in a kneeling position with shins and top of feet on the floor, hands resting calmly on knees) then bring your arms back and grab onto your foot soles. Bring your chin to your chest and round your back and body forward, folding your body at the pelvis. When doing this, your head should come down towards the floor and your forehead should touch your knees. Bring your hips up a small amount as the top of your head touches the floor. Inhale five deeps breathes as you comfortably hold this position, then go back into your hero pose. Do this several times for the best effect.

The cobra pose, also known as 'Bhujangasana' is another simple yet effective pose that is good for hormone regulation. Specifically, the cobra pose is good for massaging the adrenal glands. Helping the adrenal gland function better can aid in helping your body to better fight stress and let go of tension easier. Start the cobra pose by lying flat on your belly with legs together and your hands on the floor even with your shoulders. Start with your forehead resting flat on the floor. Then simply lift your head and chest upward, lengthening your spine and stretching your core. Take several deep breaths, inhaling and exhaling slowly for several seconds and then lower yourself back to the ground. Do this pose several times and take a few minutes to really appreciate and enjoy the feeling of the cobra pose and its benefits.

The third simple, yet effective yoga pose for hormone regulation is the camel pose, also known as 'Ustrasana'. The camel pose has quite a large variety of known advantages and benefits. One of them being, of course, to aid in the regulation of hormones. As the pose is being held, it helps to stimulate the internal organs and structures especially in the neck and shoulder regions of the body. As was stated earlier, this is where the thyroids glands are located, and they appear to really like the benefits of the camel pose. To begin the camel pose, start with a kneeling position. Keep your knees at the same width apart as your pelvis. Bring your thighs in towards each other and bring your pelvis forward and up towards the torso. Meanwhile, be sure you are keeping your shins and feet firmly pressed to the ground. Take your hand to the back of your hips with your palms toward your body. Push down on your tailbone area with your palms as you push your thighs back to compensate your body moving forward. Then take a big deep breathe as your shoulder blades move in the direction of your ribs. Lean backward a little bit and relax your torso and rib areas as you relax and pull your chest away from your hips. Take your hands down to your heels and move your arms out. Try and hold the position for thirty to forty-five seconds before bringing up your upper body and returning to the original position. Perform the position several times to really get the best effects and hormone affecting benefits.

The reason that yoga and Pilates can aid in being successful on your intermittent fasting journey is that it can help to control cravings and hunger, it is good exercise, and most importantly, it helps with the hormonal balancing. A large part of what makes intermittent fasting beneficial and why women are seeing such great results with it is that it is helping to naturally regulate the body's hormones to better acclimate it to a faster and more efficient metabolism. So while yoga has great benefits for the mind, body, and soul, it is also great for natural hormonal regulation!

Cardio — Running, Cycling, and Swimming to Help with Intermittent Fasting Results

There was a myth going around for a while that doing cardio on an empty stomach can help with losing the 'stubborn' fat. This is false. Doing fasted cardio is actually what helps to lose those stubborn fat places. To define what exactly cardiovascular exercise is, it is an aerobic exercise that uses oxygen to meet the demands of energy during exercising. Examples of cardio workouts are swimming, running, cycling — basically any aerobic type activity. This basically means it is an exercise that specifically works the heart, the lungs, and that oxygen intake is required to participate in.

To break it all down, cardio done in a fed state is not quite as effective as cardio performed in a fasted state. The difference between an empty stomach and a fasted state is essentially when you do your cardio. If you do your cardio in your feeding window, you are not in the fasted state of lowered insulin and blood sugar and your body is working on processing the foods you have been feeding it in your eating window. While generally any exercise burns energy and helps you to lose weight no matter what your insulin levels are at, there are some pretty specific benefits of doing your cardio in a fasted state. One of the subtle benefits of doing cardio in a fasted state is that lipolysis and fat oxidation rates are increased.

Basically, lipolysis is the breaking down of fat cells by the body to use as energy. Essentially, this means to enter a fat burning state. Fat oxidation simply means the burning of this energy by the cells. So cardio exercise helps the body to break down and burn fat stores easier in a fasted state. The claims of fasted cardio helping with 'stubborn belly fat' stem from the studies that show increased blood flow to the stomach and abdominal reasons in the state of a fast. With minimal blood flow to a certain area or region of the body, it means less fat

140

burning chemicals and therefore there is a less fat loss to certain areas of the body with less blood flow.

Fasted cardio is a bit of a double-edged sword in the sense that there are a few downsides to it. There is some evidence that fasted cardio can cause some muscle breakdown as well. While this generally is not catastrophic or really, all that significant, it can have an effect. This is not ideal because if you break down enough muscle too quickly. Your body will not be able to keep up with the repairs required to build more muscle and could eventually actually lead to muscle loss. Ultimately fasted cardio to aid with weight loss and overall health is more beneficial than not. But as mentioned, it does come with a couple of risks and should be used with care and caution. Cardio is generally great for cardiac health and stamina, regardless of what diet plan or routine you are on.

Strength Training and Intermittent Fasting

Strength training combined with intermittent fasting and healthy eating can provide some truly great results. Strength training, also known as weight lifting or resistance training is anaerobic exercise based off using resistance to cause muscle contraction, which in turn builds muscle, improves anaerobic endurance and enlarges the size of the skeletal muscles.

Many people believe that strength training is more beneficial than cardio of exercise when combining it with intermittent fasting. The theory is that it is an ideal way to maintain lean body mass is by intermittent fasting and strength training regularly as well as following a high protein low carb diet. Many women see great results combining these things.

Resistance training is more for building muscle than burning fat but is also excellent for maintaining the lean body mass. Doing strength training during the fasted state is typically giving the best results. If

141

you do resistance training during a feeding period, keep in mind that your body is working on other things like digesting food and re-acclimating to the feeding period. Many women have said they have more energy and feel they have more effective workouts when performing their resistance training during a fast, as they are hyper-focused on the task at hand. Ultimately, strength training is an excellent addition to the intermittent fasting lifestyle and many women are achieving excellent results.

Meditation and Mindfulness

Meditation can be an excellent tool for focus, clearing the mind and aiding in success with any lifestyle change, especially intermittent fasting. It is an ancient technique that helps to focus and clear the mind. Meditation actually changes the structure of the brain and allows it to be clear and promote simple clear thoughts. It can give you almost superhuman abilities like being able to keep a calm clear head in a high-pressure situation and use the power of the mind to your advantage.

In the last ten years, scientists have discovered that every time we think or learn something, new a neuro connection appears in the brain. The neuro connections we use the most frequently, like a habit or routine, grow stronger with each use and weaker over time they are not in use until they eventually disappear. This is why certain habits are completely automatic. These are the same reasons that meditation is exceptionally useful for starting and using intermittent fasting. It helps to reinforce the habits necessary to be successful and to embed them in the brain. When you first begin to fast, it is often said how difficult the first few days are. Meditation can really help to clear the mind and allow you to focus on the challenge at hand. Usually, this is overcoming your hunger. Many women use meditation to get through the first stages of hunger and it really helps to reduce their stress, hanger, and hanxiety while your body adjusts to you first several fasting periods.

When and if you first decide to give meditation a try, there are several steps and techniques that you can follow to have a successful meditation. Start with finding a quiet atmosphere where you are either alone or a place that you are able to relax and clear your mind. Choose loose fitting and comfortable clothes for your meditation session, it is important to be comfortable and relaxed. Keep in mind that you will need to sit the whole time so wear something that is comfortable for that. Doing pre-meditating yoga and or stretches is recommended especially focusing on the back and neck as these are the places that we tend to hold stress in the most. Once you have found a place, outfit and time that is suitable for your meditation you can begin. A basic position is either sitting cross-legged or in the 'lotus' position which is cross-legged with the soles of your feet pointing upward. If you have difficulty with either of these positions, just sit as comfortably as you can. Begin by closing your eyes and focusing on your breathing, focus on your inspirations and expirations while attempting to let your other thoughts fall away. Do not try to control your breathing and try not to focus on anything else. When first starting out, only meditate for five to seven minutes a day.

When you are incorporating meditation with intermittent fasting, begin doing it when you start to feel initial pangs of hunger that you feel you cannot ignore. After you meditate, you should feel calm and relaxed and with luck, it will help to distract you from your hunger. It is ideal to meditate at the same time every day. Your body likes routine and it will begin to expect meditation at a certain time. People that are experienced in meditation can do it for up to twenty to thirty minutes a day. Practicing meditation is a great way to help you to overcome hunger, focus on your daily important tasks, and prepare your mind for a fast. There are many great resources available for free online to help you with practicing meditation.

Combining Intermittent Fasting with Other Diets

Since intermittent fasting is not really a diet, it is a pattern of feeding and fasting, and many women combine it with other diet plans. Intermittent fasting goes along great with other diets and women are getting great results. Intermittent fasting is compatible with many diets because it is adjustable and based less off of what is being consumed and more of when food is being consumed. The most popular diets that intermittent fasting is combined with is the ketogenic diet, the gluten-free diet, the paleo diet, and a vegan diet.

Combining Intermittent Fasting with a Ketogenic Diet

As many people already know, ketogenic diets have become exceptionally popular in the past several years. Combining both a keto diet and an intermittent fasting lifestyle is probably the best, quickest, and most effective way to lose weight. The keto diet is incredibly popular because it is so effective, especially in women. The keto diet is based on a high fat, low carb, and moderate protein type of protocol. Combining a keto diet with intermittent fasting can be extremely beneficial and productive, especially for weight loss and overall health.

The theory behind a ketogenic diet is that you achieve ketosis which is a stable level of blood sugar. The keto diet is based on high fat because fat is one of the first sources of fuel that your body converts into energy when consumed. By feeding your body high in healthy fat foods, it helps it to be more efficient in the breakdown. There are numerous benefits to combining intermittent fasting with a ketogenic diet; you will get very few cravings for starters. One of the desirable effects of the ketogenic diet is that it is exceptional at stabilizing blood sugar. Since keto is fat based, you will not get spikes in your blood sugar and therefore your insulin will not rise and give you food cravings. A ketogenic diet already is known for suppressing hunger.

When you are on a ketogenic diet, it encourages the liver to produce more keynotes. The ketones get into your bloodstream and the cells use them as fuel. Ketones also are known for suppressing ghrelin, the body's hormone that tells you when to eat. With the ketogenic diet already suppressing your hunger, fasting comes significantly easier and allows you to fast in longer windows and get the benefits of a longer fast.

Fat loss is another excellent benefit to combining the two diets. Both intermittent fasting and the keto diet increase fat loss, even without calorie restriction. Together the two eating styles create a superhuman fat burning machine. Many women drop weight swiftly and because the ghrelin hormone has already been suppressed, you do not feel nearly as deprived and hungry as you would with a traditional diet plan.

Ketosis

When hearing about a ketogenic diet, the term ketosis also come up. At one point, it was thought that being in a state of ketosis was bad for you. However, the ketogenic diet is based on being in a state of ketosis, this is actually the goal. Ketosis is a state in which the metabolism achieved where there are heightened ketones in the bloodstream and body tissues. It is a state of naturally lowered insulin. Ketones are water-soluble protein bodies that are produced by the liver from fatty acids during periods of low food intake or carb restricted diets. Ketosis helps the body to transition to a state of fat burning. When in ketosis, you will unlikely feel very hungry because your insulin is naturally lowered. Ketosis is the goal for following a ketogenic diet as it is the state in which the body is burning stored fat. In the fat burning state is when the most weight loss occurs.

Keto flu

Many women that live a keto lifestyle are familiar with the term 'keto flu.' This is basically your body's reaction to taking away its carbs. When you stop your carb intake, your body is no longer using carbs as its primary fuel source. When you are no longer using carbs for fuel, your body enters a state of ketosis, which is when it switches to burning fat. The symptoms come from your body adjusting to running off ketones. Ketones are what your liver produces during periods of fasting or starvation and are by-products of fat breakdown.

Many people really struggle with the lack of carbs and show symptoms within just a day or two. Symptoms can range in severity, some being mild to non-existent and others lasting longer. The average length of keto flu is about a week. Symptoms include nausea, vomiting, constipation, poor concentration, lack of energy, stomach pain, dizziness, weakness, irritability, muscle soreness, sugar cravings, and difficulties sleeping. To combat the keto flu, it is important to stay well hydrated and get enough sleep. Other ways to help combat the keto flu include getting enough electrolytes, avoiding excessive exercise, avoiding ambient light, and getting enough fat in your diet.

Taking good care of yourself during the first few days of transitioning to keto and fasting is essential in staying healthy. Be sure to plan your eating and meals ahead of time. Many women do a slow step down from carbs instead of going cold turkey to help avoid the keto flu. Cutting out just a few carbs each day and adding more fat is a common technique to adjust the body to the change. You still may get symptoms of the keto flu, but it may help them be less severe. It is also a good idea to switch either to keto or intermittent fasting first. Sometimes doing them both together can be too much stress on your body at once. Adapting to intermittent fasting first will help with one change at a time. Not everyone gets the keto flu, but do not be alarmed if you do.

As with most unpleasant things, it will pass, and you can hurry it along with supportive care for yourself.

Combining Intermittent Fasting with a Vegan Diet

Combining intermittent fasting with a vegan diet can be a greater challenge as vegan or plant-based food does not have healthy fats as readily available as animal-based foods. Having said that, it is not impossible and can still be conducive with the lifestyle of intermittent fasting. Basically, the difference between eating a regular diet and eating a vegan diet is that vegans do not eat any animal-based foods. They strictly eat plant-based foods and fruits, vegetables and substitutes like tofu etc. What makes combining veganism with intermittent fasting difficult the lack of natural fats available. When your body enters a fat burning state, it is more difficult to break a fast without any animal-based product. It is not impossible though and many vegans have had luck with it. Like with any diet, there are loopholes and ways to make it work with your lifestyle. Many vegans simply just have to eat more carbs. Nuts and seeds are good sources of protein and fat and are popular in a vegan diet in general.

Ultimately, since intermittent fasting is not exactly a diet as opposed to a pattern of eating, you technically do not need to change and supplement the vegan diet. While veganism can have excellent health benefits, it can be a struggle to get all the proper nutrition without an animal-based diet. The human body was designed to break down and ingest animal-based fats and food so training it to live off of plant-based foods can be a challenge. Most vegans will need to supplement with vitamins and minerals to meet all the health needs. Ultimately though, it is possible to live and remain healthy on a vegan diet along with engaging in intermittent fasting.

Humans are omnivores and should be able to adequately adjust to sole plant-based diets as long as they are properly supplemented. When beginning intermittent fasting with your vegan lifestyle, it is always a good idea to get advice or consult with your regular physician to find out the best and healthiest ways to safely participate.

Combining with a Paleo Diet

Combining intermittent fasting with a paleo diet is about as simple as you can get. Basically, a paleo diet is a diet based off what food was consumed during the stone ages and ancient times. When there were no stores, supermarkets, delis, and fast food restaurants, what was left? There were plants, meats, berries, vegetables, and whatever food could be hunted, picked, made or gathered.

Back in stone age times, when paleo eating was the only available way of life, intermittent fasting was already part of the lifestyle. It was part of life because food just was not always available. So, paleo diets are quite simple and go well with intermittent fasting. If you were to pretend you were living in ancient-paleo times, you would already be participating in intermittent fasting because that was a natural part of life in those days. Depending on where you lived, there were winters and food was not always available to be picked and gathered. Animals moved south, and hunting became scarce. So, what did you do when there was no food to be found? You simply did not eat, and your body adapted until you could.

In recent popular culture, the paleo diet has been enormously helpful in helping women with weight-loss and engaging in a natural basic diet by simply cutting out process food, carbs, and anything with preservatives. The paleo diet strips it all down to the basics of the human needs for food. A diet that simply involves protein, fruits, and vegetables. Combining this diet with intermittent fasting and some regular exercise can and will result in excellent results as far as feeling better and more energized and with weight loss.

The Gluten-Free Diet and Intermittent Fasting

Many people have seen the effects and benefits of going gluten-free. People with digestive and stomach issues often change to gluten-free. Gluten-free goes just as well with intermittent fasting as any other diet. It is important to keep an eye on your caloric intake as gluten-free diets often are carb free as well. Gluten-free diets tend to have a lot of foods that contain a lot of flour, so watch out for the carb count when eating gluten-free. Many women that are gluten-free already have good grasps of what goes well with their diet and where they can find foods that work for them. Adding in the timed fasting is just one step further that can take you closer to your goals and help to lead to a better and healthier life.

Essential Oils to Help with Intermittent Fasting and Weight Loss

Essential oils are a rapidly growing fad and are useful for many different ailments and can provide support for multiple body systems. While the use of essential oils is controversial in their effectiveness, many women swear by them and there is some evidence they can help with weight loss as well as provide immune support as well as mental health support. The route in which to use essential oils is varied. They can be used in a diffuser, inhaled in an inhaler, rubbed on the skin, made into body wraps, burned in candles, and many more options. They work both topically and aromatically. There are five specific essential oils geared toward weight loss as well as many that help with psychological challenges.

Grapefruit Essential Oils

Grapefruit essential oils contain d-limonene, a chemical that increases the rate of the metabolism because it induces lipolysis or the breakdown of fat cells. Grapefruit essential oils also help to fight cellulite in women. Grapefruit essential oils work best as a massage oil or bath salt. Grapefruit essential oils can be used daily for best results.

Peppermint Essential Oils

Peppermint is a great oil for energy and can really help to stifle cravings. It is refreshing to smell and has positive effects when inhaled; it is a natural bronchodilator and helps improve oxygen flow. Peppermint essential oils work best when inhaled directly. Put it in a diffuser for twenty minutes a day or put several drops onto a cloth or handkerchief and inhale directly for best results.

Lemon Essential Oils

Lemon smells fantastic and is quite useful in helping to block out thoughts of greasy foods and sugar. It has properties that help to improve energy and helps to increase your mood. Lemon essential oils are great for right before a workout. It works best in a diffuser for fifteen to twenty minutes.

Rosemary Essential Oils

Rosemary has an herbal, refreshing type smell and can really help in suppressing the appetite. Rosemary can help with water retention and surpass craving as well as help with cellulite prevention. Give it a sniff when you are struggling with a certain food craving. It is also a great massage oil and is effective as a bath salt. Rosemary has other health benefits as well and can even help with menstrual-related bloating.

Ginger Essential Oils

Ginger is a powerful detox aid. Ginger has detoxifying effects that are quite helpful with purging the body and mind of cravings and toxins. Ginger also helps to stimulate the lymph nodes, and it helps to stimulate blood flow and goes great in a bath! Many women mix with coconut oil and use topically. Ginger should be used with some caution as it is a "hot" oil and can cause the feelings of burning. Mixing four to five drops of ginger essential oil and two to three tablespoons of coconut oil and adding it to your bath is a great way to reap the benefits of ginger!

Lavender Essential Oils

Lavender is perhaps the most popular and well-known essential oil. Probably because it has such a diverse range of uses and effects. Lavender's best known for its calming properties. These are especially useful for when and if you experience 'hanger' or anxiety during a fast. Lavender helps to calm the irritability. Lavender is also a good sleep aid and can be used in a variety of forms. It can be applied topically, inhaled or ingested.

While essential oils certainly are not for everyone, they can and do help many women to overcome struggles both with intermittent fasting and wit weight loss in general. Sometimes, a sniff of the right oil is all you need to get over the hurdle at hand, whether it is to maintain a fast or get past a craving. The first few days of a fast or diet are always the most difficult and any support you can get is usually worth considering. They certainly have a place in a healthy life if you are willing to give them a try.

The Buddy System

Having a friend to endeavor into the intermittent fasting lifestyle with can make all the difference. For any life change, it is important to have a strong support system, you want to have someone to bounce off ideas, questions, and concerns with. Ask your friends and family if they are interested in a healthier lifestyle and find someone to do it with you. If no one you know personally is interested, there are various great blogs, discussion groups, and social media pages specifically for people that want to participate in the intermittent fasting and healthy eating lifestyle. Having a friend or support system to lean on especially when getting through your first few fast where your body is still adjusting to the new pattern can really make all the difference in success. There are also podcasts and talk shows that have great info about personal struggles and successes while intermittently fasting. Be sure to have a solid support system before beginning intermittent fasting.

Supplements and Vitamins to Aid in Fasting

Getting adequate vitamins and proper nutrition is absolutely vital while doing the intermittent fasting lifestyle. It is especially important because intermittent fasting is essentially forcing your body into a state of fat burning. In a state of fat burning, you are also in ketosis typically. Taking supplemental vitamins may be necessary during your fasting periods, especially if you are engaging in a long-term fast. Most multivitamins will due, but it is important to know what is in them and what they should contain to aid with your fast.

Sodium and Potassium

Levels of ketones in the bloodstream rise during your periods of fasting which cause your body to signal a flushing response. This quickly depletes the stores of potassium and sodium. It can cause fatigue, low energy, and the feeling of being lightheaded. These minerals are very important for ketogenesis and without them, the body really must work and struggle to access the stores of fat.

Magnesium

Magnesium is a body mineral that regulates several vital body functions. Magnesium helps to regulate nerve and blood pressure and is easily and swiftly depleted in the period of fasting. Low magnesium is what can cause the feeling of brain fogginess or muscle cramps during a fasting period.

B-Complex Vitamins

B-complex vitamin, which includes riboflavin, niacin, thiamine, and biotin are vitamins that aid the body in absorbing nutrients. B-complex vitamins do not get flushed out of the body in the same way sodium, potassium, and magnesium does during the state of ketosis. However, there are a large number of women that are chronically low or have B-complex vitamin deficiencies.

Vitamin D

Vitamin D is a very common deficiency amongst both men and women. Vitamin D is rather difficult to obtain through food intake and is acquired naturally through sunlight. Vitamin D is vital to both immune health and bone density. Vitamin D helps the use nutrients that are critical to body functions and helps allow the nutrients to function, magnesium being one of them.

Chromium

Chromium is not as common in your everyday multivitamin but there has been some research that shows it can be a culprit that mitigates hunger. This can be problematic as it may force you to end your fast earlier than planned or expected due to the hunger pangs.

Beta-Hydroxybutyrate or BHB

Many women who intermittently fast also take a BHB supplement as well, these are also known as exogenous ketones. This means ketones that are not produced by the body. One of the three ketone bodies is BHB. Ketone bodies are what is naturally produced by the liver when you are in a state of ketosis. If broken down to the cellular level, the human body needs BHB to access and adequately use the fat stores for energy. Using a BHB supplement during a fast helps to ensure that the body will have the necessary levels of BHB in the bloodstream.

Having the proper levels of BHB in the bloodstream will help to facilitate the metabolizing of fat into energy.

Branched Chain Amino Acids

Branched-chain amino acids are amino acids that produce the same important amino acids that are found in protein. These amino acids allow the body to not only help build muscle but also to help sustain it. The downside to Branch Chain Amino Acid supplements is that they do contain a few calories, something around six calories per gram and could potentially disrupt a fast to a certain extent. Most people take Branch Chain Amino Acid supplements when they are working on strength training and building muscle as part of their daily routine. While many people have good positive effects with this supplement and experience no negative impact, this is not always the case and if having a strictly caloric free fast is important to you personally, this may be a supplement to avoid.

Water (H2O)

Drinking water is absolutely vital to any and all diets and fasts. This cannot be stressed enough. Lack of hydration is often the biggest factor in nearly all negative side effects to any fast. Body organs and tissues including the brain depend and utilize water to maintain the proper levels of nutrients, vitamins, and minerals. Dehydration has a wide variety of symptoms and can quickly lead to fatigue, irritability, dizziness, confusion, headache, and many other symptoms and feelings of discomfort. Maintaining proper hydration throughout a fast is important and allows any supplemental vitamins to work better.

Ultimately, taking a good multivitamin during a fast can significantly help your body systems out and help your fast be just a little bit easier. Taking proper supplementation can aid in muscle building and help to improve the positive benefits of the fasting lifestyle. Choose a vitamin that contains what was just covered and you will be able to reap the benefits a little bit easier.

Alcohol and Intermittent Fasting

Many women enjoy having a beer or margarita after a long day, socially, or just for fun. The trouble with drinking while fasting is that there are calories in an alcoholic drink. Depending on what hours you are eating and fasting, you will need to plan to drink only during feeding periods. Drinking will break a fast. As far as healthier options with alcohol, low-calorie drinks are ideal, beer tends to be high in carbs. There are various recipes for 'skinny' margaritas and martinis. There are even low carb beers available. The most important things to remember with all intermittent fasting protocols is that when you eat is always more important than what you eat. Keeping yourself well hydrated is important to any diet, but it is especially important to an intermittent fasting diet plan which makes it even more important if you choose to drink while in an intermittent fasting program.

Pop or Soda and Intermittent Fasting

Drinking pop on a fast will without a doubt bring your fast to a screeching halt. Pop is high in sugar and chemicals that your body can really struggle with breaking down. Even diet pops are not particularly good. They are hard on the digestive system and can be corrosive to the gut lining. If you are a pop-acholic, it may be best to consider giving it up or at the very least switching to diet pop. Try and avoid even diet pop during a fast and especially regular pop as it will immediately reverse to the state of ketosis. Many women found they had weight losses simply by cutting pop out of their daily diet.

Chapter Six

While it has been mentioned several times that intermittent fasting is more of a lifestyle as opposed to a diet, there are certain recipes and eating patterns that can aid in intermittent fasting. Certain meals and eating patterns can help to bring out and encourage the benefits of intermittent fasting. Below are several examples that are simple and easy to make that work nicely with an intermittent fasting program. Several of the recipes are both keto-based and gluten-free. There are lots of great options for healthy delicious meals that are easy to prepare!

Three Simple and Easy Recipes for Breakfast

The Caprese Omelet — Healthy and Low-Carb

The healthy, low carb Caprese Omelet is easy and a good vegetarian option (not vegan though).

It can be made in just minutes and is an excellent filler. It is great with either store bought or homemade pesto.

- o Three large eggs
- o One tbsp. of butter or ghee
- o One-third of a cup of cherry tomatoes, cut in half
- o Two slices fresh mozzarella cheese
- o Three to six basil leaves, chopped up well
- o One heaped tbsp. grated parmesan cheese
- o One tbsp. pesto
- o Sea salt and pepper, or to taste
- o Additional Option: One tsp. of balsamic vinegar and one tbsp. extra virgin olive oil to drizzle on top of the omelet

The Instructions: Combine ingredients together in a bowl, be sure to mix well. Use a medium pan and add a little butter and melt. Pour mixture in and heat until the egg is cooked on one side. Then fold omelet in half and cook both sides until done. Drizzle balsamic vinegar and olive oil if desired.

The Super Electrolyte Smoothie and Cereal

This smoothie and cereal are a great breakfast, snack, or evening meal that is both delicious, simple to make, and great for keeping yourself on a healthy track. While these are keto diet based, they are still great breakfast options. They are both quick and easy to prepare with easy to find ingredients.

Super Electrolyte Smoothie:

- One-half of a large avocado or three and a half ounces
- One-half of a cup of coconut milk such as Aroy-D or four fluid ounces
- One-third of a cup of frozen mixed berries or one and a half ounces
- One and a half cups unsweetened almond milk or cashew milk or twelve fluid ounces
- One tbsp. raw cacao powder or a quarter of an ounce
- One-fourth of a tsp. cinnamon
- One-fourth of a tsp. vanilla bean powder
- Two tbsp. of collagen powder or half an ounce

The Instructions: Blend well in a blender until smooth and pourable, then pour into a glass to enjoy.

Super Cereal (Keto-Based)

- One-fourth of a cup flaked almonds or twenty-three grams
- One-fourth of a cup unsweetened flaked coconut or fifteen grams
- One-fourth of a tsp. of cinnamon powder
- One tsp. of virgin coconut oil
- Toppings:

- Two tbsp. of cacao nibs or one ounce
- Two tbsp. of hemp seeds or three-quarters of an ounce
- Optional: Fresh or frozen berries for the top

The Instructions: Add to a bowl and add fresh or frozen berries to the top.

Low-Carb Porridge – Anti-Inflammatory

This is a great warm breakfast, especially for the winter. It is unique because it contains some beneficial supplements such as turmeric (a spice that helps our body adapt to changes), and bee pollen (bee pollen has immune boosting properties and natural anti-inflammatory properties). If you are dealing with any kind of chronic pain or inflammation, this is an ideal meal for you.

- Two tbsp. of hemp seeds
- One-fourth of a cup of walnut or pecan halves
- One-fourth of a cup of unsweetened toasted coconut
- Two tbsp. of whole chia seeds
- Three-fourths of a cup of unsweetened almond milk
- One-fourth of a cup of coconut milk
- One-fourth of a cup of almond butter, preferably roasted
- One tbsp. extra virgin coconut oil or MCT oil or fifteen milliliters
- One-fourth to one half of a cup of ground turmeric or one half to one tsp. freshly grated turmeric
- One tsp. bee pollen or one-half tsp. cinnamon or one-half tsp. vanilla powder
- Pinch ground black pepper (significantly helps to improves turmeric absorption in the bloodstream)
- Optional: Two tbsp. Erythritol or Swerve or five to ten drops liquid stevia (NuNaturals or Sweet Leaf brands are ideal brands to use for this recipe)

Three Simple and Easy Recipes for Lunch

The Five-Minute Quick and Healthy Tuna Salad

This meal is easy to make and is full of superfoods, high in the good fats, and protein. This is ideal for lunch, after a workout, or for coming out of a fast. Tuna is a great lean protein and eggs are a good fat blast. Enjoy this tuna salad for lunch or for dinner.

- o One-fourth of a cup of mayonnaise - Paleo mayonnaise is preferred
- o One tbsp. of lemon juice or fifteen milliliters
- o Two tbsp. of olive oil- extra virgin
- o One tbsp. parsley or chives- chopped
- o One-fourth of a tsp. each pepper and salt, or to taste
- o One medium head of romaine lettuce
- o One-half of a sliced small yellow or red onion
- o One medium cucumber or four to five gherkins
- o Eight sliced large olives
- o One drained jar of tuna- large
- o Four hard-boiled eggs- large

The Instructions: Combine the mayonnaise, parsley, onion, lemon juice, olive oil, and tuna in a bowl and mix well. Use the head of lettuce to make a lettuce bed and add tuna mixture to the top. Add the sliced hard-boiled eggs, olives, and cucumbers to the top. Serve and enjoy!

The All-Day Mexican Salad Bowl

This simple, delicious, and easy to make Mexican recipe is quick and packed full of healthy fats. This Mexican bowl is a great choice for helping to break a fast as it high in healthy fats that will help to keep your insulin levels stable. This Mexican bowl is quick and ideal for any time of the day!

- o Two Mexican chorizo sausages

- o Two gluten-free Italian style sausages
- o One-half of a jalapeno pepper
- o One tbsp. of fresh oregano or one tsp. dried oregano
- o One small yellow onion, diced
- o One-half of a cup of halved cherry tomatoes
- o One-half of a red bell pepper, chopped well
- o One medium spring onion, sliced well
- o One tbsp. extra virgin olive oil or fifteen milliliters
- o One-fourth of a tsp. of coconut aminos
- o One tsp. of fresh lime juice
- o One tbsp. of chopped and fresh coriander
- o Two large eggs
- o One-half of a large avocado, sliced
- o One-fourth of a tsp. of paprika
- o Salt and pepper to taste

Instructions: Cook sausage separately and add to salad, combine all ingredient, and enjoy!

Three Simple and Easy Recipes for Dinner

Green Chicken Chile Cauliflower Casserole

This is a relatively simple and quick dish to make that is both great for a keto diet and can be adapted to a gluten-free diet as well.

- o One pound or four hundred and fifty grams of ground beef, turkey, chicken, or pork (chicken is most commonly used and the easiest)
- o Two tablespoons butter
- o Three-fourths of a cup of chopped onion
- o Three-fourths of a cup of a chopped celery stalk
- o Two and a half cups of cauliflower rice
- o One cup of shredded Monterrey Jack cheese, or mozzarella cheese

- o   One cup of shredded sharp cheddar cheese
- o   One-half of a cup of chicken or vegetable broth
- o   Four ounces of canned green chiles - be sure to drain
- o   One-half of a cup of sour cream, full-fat variety
- o   One-half of a teaspoon of garlic powder
- o   One-half of a cup of softened cream cheese
- o   Salt and fresh cracked black pepper
- o   Cilantro - add as a garnish on top

Instructions for Baking: Preheat oven to 325 degrees, cook rice according to the details on the package, and once cooked, drain and set aside. Melt butter in a medium-sized pan over medium heat, add the ground meat of your choice and cook for five to seven minutes. Then add the onion and celery and cook for an additional five minutes, and then add salt and pepper to taste. Get a large bowl and add the rice, add the cheese, chiles, sour cream, cream cheese, the meat and veggie mix, and the stock. Also, add the garlic powder and black pepper. Spread the mix out evenly in the baking pan and top off with the leftover cheese. Then proceed to bake at 325 degrees for twenty to twenty-five minutes or until cheese is nice and bubbling. Add the cilantro to garnish and enjoy this simple and delicious meal!

Garlic Butter Chicken Bites with Zucchini Noodles

This is another quick meal to produce that is popular and tasty. It fits in well to most diets even though it is technically a keto meal.

- o   Three to four boneless and skinless chicken breasts, cut into medium bite-sized chunks
- o   Four to five medium zucchinis, rinsed and spiralized (or a pack of Zucchini Noodles that you bought at the store)
- o   Four tablespoons butter, divided up
- o   Two teaspoons of minced garlic
- o   One tablespoon of hot sauce - brands may vary

- One-fourth of a cup or sixty milliliters of low sodium chicken broth- bone broth can also be used
- Juice of one half of a lemon
- One tablespoon of minced parsley
- One teaspoon of fresh thyme leaves
- Crushed red chili pepper flakes- option
- Several slices of lemon to use for garnish
- The Marinade
- Two tablespoons of olive oil
- One tablespoon of hot sauce (Sriracha is popular but other brands can be used) or one teaspoon of chili powder
- Two teaspoons of salt
- One teaspoon of fresh cracked black pepper
- Two teaspoons of garlic powder
- One teaspoon of Italian seasoning

Instructions: Cut up the chicken breast into bite-sized pieces and combine with olive oil, pepper, garlic powder, salt, Italian seasoning, chili powder or hot sauce and mix up well in a bowl until it is seasoned evenly, then allow to marinate in the fridge for a half to one hour. Wash zucchini and then use a spiralizer to make the zucchini noodles and then set them aside. Set out the chicken pieces in marinade until they reach room temperature. Stir fry the chicken pieces until they are a golden brown and then remove and set aside. In the same pan over high heat, add two tablespoons of butter, lemon juice, and the hot sauce. Let it simmer and reduce for one to two minutes while stirring regularly. Stir in the minced garlic and fresh parsley and then add in the zucchini noodles. Allow the juices to reduce for a minute if the juice from the zucchini gives out too much water. Finally, add the chicken bites back into the pan and stir for another minute or two to reheat. Add more parsley for garnish along with crushed chili pepper, lemon slices, and fresh thyme. This dish is best if served immediately.

Buttery Garlic Herb Chicken with Lemon Cauliflower Rice

This dish is popular and both keto-friendly and gluten-free. A low-carb dish that is easy and can be made quickly and that the whole family can enjoy.

o One and a half pounds (six hundred and fifty grams) of boneless skinless chicken thighs or breasts
o Two tablespoons of butter
o One teaspoon of chopped fresh thyme and one teaspoon of fresh chopped oregano, one teaspoon of freshly chopped rosemary
o Fourteen ounces of (four hundred grams) of cauliflower rice (one medium head)
o One medium onion, chopped well
o Four garlic cloves, minced well
o One-fourth of a cup (sixty milliliters) of chicken broth
o One tablespoon of hot sauce
o One-half of a cup of grated parmesan cheese
o One-half of a cup fresh chopped parsley
o Juice of one half of a lemon, add zest, and lemon slices for garnishing
o The marinade
o One teaspoon of Italian seasoning
o One tablespoon olive oil
o One teaspoon paprika
o Fresh cracked pepper, to taste
o Juice of one half of a lemon

The Instructions: In a big bowl, set chicken thighs and sprinkle with paprika, Italian seasoning, olive oil, black pepper, and lemon juice. Mix together well and allow to marinate for ten to fifteen minutes. Meanwhile, put the cauliflower florets on pulse in a food processor for about fifteen to thirty seconds or until you obtain a rice-like consistency. Then set this aside for now.

163

Melt two tablespoons of butter in a medium-sized pan over medium to low heat. Then add the oregano, thyme, and the rosemary. Set the chicken with the skin side down and cook for four to five minutes on each side until the chicken is no longer pink in color and reaches 165°F in temperature. Cooking time will vary a little depending on the size of the chicken thighs. Remove chicken from the pan and set aside. Keep the cooking juices from the chicken thighs and fat in the pan for now. Using the same pan, fry the garlic and the onion for one minute until fragrant but be sure not to burn it. Add in the hot sauce and stir to mix well. Then add the riced cauliflower and mix everything else together. Add in the chicken stock, the parsley, the lemon zest, and lemon juice. Cook for two or three minutes to reduce cooking juices then put in the parmesan cheese. Then proceed to adjust seasoning as it is needed. Put the chicken thighs over cauliflower rice and reheat in a swift fashion. Serve with the fresh, cracked black pepper, red chili pepper flakes, fresh herbs, and more parmesan if you want.

Along with a teaspoon of fresh thyme, be sure it is chopped well.

Super Foods and Intermittent Fasting

Superfoods have certainly been an ongoing rage in the last few years or so, and many of them rightly deserve the title! There are many great foods that go along great with the intermittent fasting lifestyle and several super foods that are particularly useful in aiding with overall health and weight loss. A superfood is considered a food that is very rich in vitamins and minerals and has extra benefits as opposed to a regular food. Some of these superfoods can and will really help you out when you are in your feeding period, as well as overall health and longevity.

Superfood One: Leafy Dark Greens

Dark leafy greens are rich in nutrients, zinc, calcium, iron, and folate just to name a few. What really makes dark leafy greens in the 'super'

164

category is that it has the potential to drastically reduce the risk of certain diseases including type two diabetes and heart disease. Dark leafy greens also contain high levels of anti-inflammatory properties and can actually help to prevent and fight cancer.

Superfood Two: Eggs

Eggs are also a great food that has countless health benefits. High in healthy fat and a great source of protein. They are rich in antioxidants, especially lutein and zeaxanthin. These particular antioxidants collect around the retina of the eye and help protect the eyes from sunlight and macular degeneration. Eggs are also considered one of the most nutrient-rich foods on the planet. They are also rich in phosphorus, selenium, and iron. While they do have cholesterol, it is actually the 'good' cholesterol and helps to lower and consolidate the bad cholesterol in the veins. Interestingly enough, nearly all of the nutrients in eggs are in the yolk. Eggs are a great addition to nearly all diets and go well with the intermittent fasting lifestyle.

Superfood Three: Avocado

Avocados, a beloved, delicious, and incredible superfood. It is a great substitute, great on or with many foods, and a very healthy superfood. It is considered a fruit that is greasy; the grease coming from omega 3 fatty acids which helps break down cholesterol. This is also high in fiber, vitamin D, and folic acid. It has properties to help prevent cataracts and aid with proper digestion. Avocados help to slow down aging and are high in potassium. Basically, there is little not to love about avocados, they are very healthy, go with just about everything and are loaded with good, healthy greases, and antioxidants. The avocado goes great with intermittent fasting. Many people use avocados when breaking a fast or easing back into eating. They have a tough outer skin with a smooth inside and can be spread on food, scooped, and eaten or made into something. Avocados are excellent for health in general.

Superfood Four: Turmeric

Exceptionally popular in the last five or so years. Turmeric has gotten quite the magical reputation. While it is not an end all cure all, it is a superfood with plenty of positive health effects. Turmeric is actually a spice from India that has been used for medicinal purposes of several hundred years. Turmeric has powerful antioxidants and a solid anti-inflammatory property. The downside of turmeric is that it does not absorb into the bloodstream particularly well; however, using black pepper, another spice, does help with that. Since turmeric does not absorb well, it works better against inflammation that is more acute than chronic. Turmeric is a spice and can be used to season or mixed with other foods to get the effects and flavor. Many people that experience daily pain consume turmeric, and it fits in well with many foods and is a great natural supplement. Green tea can help to prevent damage to DNA; it is also able to shut down a specific molecule that has a role in the formation of cancer cells.

Superfood Five: Green tea

Green tea is especially great for the intermittent fasting lifestyle. The tea leaves are steamed which make them high in antioxidants. Green tea can actually help to prevent cancer, in several ways. With females that drink tea, it can help to prevent osteoporosis. Green tea helps to repair damage caused by the liver from alcohol as well. It helps prevent autoimmune disorders, Parkinson's disease, and Alzheimer's. Green tea also has caffeine which is a low-level stimulant and can increase focus. Green tea works very well in an intermittent fasting diet plan because it can be consumed at any time. It does not matter if you are in a fasting period or not. Green tea can be consumed at any point and many women have said how it really helps to get over the hunger periods and ease the transition.

According to studies in Japan, where they are big green tea drinkers, three cups of green tea a day can help to ward off breast cancer and five cups a day and you are up to sixteen percent less likely to develop heart disease. For those dedicated tea drinkers that drink at all hours of the day, decaffeinated version of green tea is also available. Green tea comes in a huge variety of flavors and beneficial to your health no matter if you prefer to drink it hot or cold. For those that are seeking the benefits of green tea but do not like the taste, there are pill forms as well.

Superfood Six: Berries

Berries are a tasty and diverse superfood. Nearly all berries are powerful antioxidants and full of fiber. Usually, the different colors mean they are rich in different vitamins. Blackberries have the highest folate levels with raspberries right behind them. Strawberries are very high in vitamins K and C. Of all the berries, raspberries have the highest fiber count. Nearly all berries are considered superfoods and have good benefits. Berries go great in smoothies, on top of cereal or oatmeal, and can be mixed and blended with many different meals. A great overall healthy food that easily works into a healthy diet.

Conclusion

In conclusion of this guide, we hope that you have learned some of the benefits and have a better understanding of how intermittent fasting, in some form or another, can be beneficial to nearly every woman. The various intermittent fasting methods have been proven to help with many health issues and weight loss, a problem that plagues thousands of women in today's society. There is evidence that is beginning to show that intermittent fasting helps to naturally regulate type two diabetes, heart health, slow down aging and countless other benefits. Every day there is more and more science-backed research showing another benefit, ranging from neurological disease prevention to the evidence that intermittent fasting could potentially help cancer patients.

The beauty of intermittent fasting is that it is more of a lifestyle as opposed to the common diet. Intermittent fasting is much less restrictive as it is focusing on when you eat more than what you eat. You can experiment with what fasting protocol best fits you and your lifestyle. Once you have adjusted to a schedule that works for you, there is nothing left but to enjoy feeling good and having the freedom to do and eat what you like. Intermittent fasting can and has helped a great variety of women to get onto the proper path for leading the healthiest life possible.

Thank you.

CPSIA information can be obtained
at www.ICGtesting.com
Printed in the USA
BVHW032211201022
649971BV00002B/3

9 781648 662089